PocketRadiologist™
Brain
Top 100 Diagnoses

PocketRadiologist™
Brain
100 Top Diagnoses

Anne G Osborn MD FACR
University Distinguished Professor of Radiology
William H and Patricia W Child Presidential Endowed Chairholder
University of Utah School of Medicine
Salt Lake City, Utah

Amersham Health Visiting Professor in Diagnostic Imaging
Armed Forces Institute of Pathology
Washington, DC

Susan I Blaser MD FRCP(C)
Neuroradiologist, The Hospital for Sick Children
Toronto, Canada

Associate Professor
The University of Toronto, Canada

Karen L Salzman MD
Assistant Professor of Radiology
Section of Neuroradiology
University of Utah School of Medicine
Salt Lake City, Utah

With 200 drawings and radiographic images

Drawings: *James A Cooper MD*
                  Lane R Bennion MS
Image Editing: *Ming Q Huang MD*
                  Melissa Petersen

AMIRSYS

W. B. SAUNDERS COMPANY
An Elsevier Science Company

AMIRSYS
A medical reference publishing company

First Edition

Text – Copyright Anne G Osborn 2002

Drawings – Copyright Amirsys Inc 2002

Compilation – Copyright Amirsys Inc 2002

Composition by Amirsys Inc, Salt Lake City, Utah

Printed by K/P Corp, Salt Lake City, Utah

ISBN: 0-7216-9708-9

Preface

The **PocketRadiologist™** series is an innovative, quick reference designed
to deliver succinct, up-to-date information to practicing professionals "at the
point of service." As close as your pocket, each title in the series is written
by world-renowned authors, specialists in their area. These experts have
designated the "top 100" diagnoses in every major body area, bulleted the
most essential facts, and offered high-resolution imaging to illustrate each
topic. Selected references are included for further review. Full color
anatomic-pathologic computer graphics model many of the actual diseases.

Each **PocketRadiologist™** title follows an identical format. The same
information is in the same place—every time—and takes you quickly from
key facts to imaging findings, differential diagnosis, pathology,
pathophysiology, and relevant clinical information.

PocketRadiologist™ titles are available in both print and hand-held PDA
formats. Our first modules feature Brain, Head and Neck, and Orthopedic
(Musculoskeletal) Imaging. Additional titles include Spine and Cord, Chest,
Breast, Vascular, Cardiac, Pediatrics, Emergency, and Genital Urinary, and
Gastro Intestinal. Enjoy!

Anne G Osborn MD
Editor-in-Chief, Amirsys Inc

PocketRadiologist™
Brain
Top 100 Diagnoses

The diagnoses in this book are divided into 11 sections in the following order:

Trauma
Infection
Aneurysms
Vascular Malformations
Stroke and Vascular Disease
Neoplasms
Cysts
Meninges
Ventricles and Cisterns
Metabolic White Matter, Degenerative Disease
Congenital Disorders

Table of Diagnoses

Neoplasms

Notice and Disclaimer

PocketRadiologist™
Brain
100 Top Diagnoses

TRAUMA

Skull Fracture (Fx)

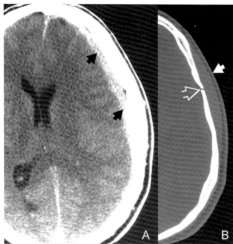

NECT scan shows acute SDH (A, black arrows) with nondisplaced linear skull fracture (B, open arrow), overlying soft tissue swelling (white arrow).

Key Facts
- Trauma = #1 cause of death/disability in young
- Skull films ineffective as trauma screen
- 1/3 of patients with severe brain injury don't have fracture (fx)
- Fxs can be linear, depressed, diastatic
- Skull base fxs can damage vessels, dura, involve cranial nerves
- Sequelae include pneumocephalus, CSF leak

Imaging Findings
General Features
- Linear fx
  - Acute fx = sharply delineated lucent line
  - Overlying soft tissue swelling almost always present
- Depressed fx
  - Fragment(s) displaced inwards
- Diastatic fx
  - Sutures spread
  - +/- Co-existing linear fx
  - May tear venous sinus, cause venous EDH
  - Cranial "burst fracture"
    - Unique in infants
    - Wide diastasis (>4mm)
    - Brain herniates through fx, extrudes under scalp
- Skull base fx
  - Can be longitudinal, transverse
  - 50% have associated intracranial mass lesion
Imaging Recommendations
- Skip the skull films
- Get NECT scan
  - Patients with high-risk mild head injury
    - GCS = 13, 14

Skull Fracture (Fx)

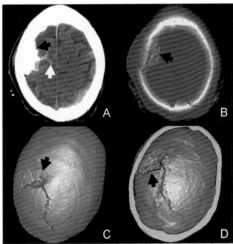

NECT scan (A, B) with 3-D reconstruction (C, D) show a comminuted, depressed anterior parietal skull fracture (black arrows). Note traumatic SAH (A, white arrow).

- ▪ 10% of patients with GCS = 15 + loss of consciousness or amnesia have abnormalities on CT scan
- ▪ 5% of patients with GCS = 15 + normal neurological exam have significant intracranial injury revealed on CT
- Use both bone, soft-tissue algorithms
- View/photograph using 3 window settings
  - ○ Soft tissue (level = 40H, window-75-100H)
  - ○ Bone (level = 500H, window = 3000H)
  - ○ Intermediate (level = 75H, window = 150-200H) to show small SDHs
- Evaluate for vascular injury if carotid canal involved

Differential Diagnosis
Suture Line
- Acute fx lucent, has sharp noncorticated margins
- Suture less distinct, has dense sclerotic borders
Vascular Groove
- Corticated margins
- Typical location (i.e., MMA)
Venous Lake
- Corticated margins
- Typical location (i.e., parasagittal)
Arachnoid Granulation
- Corticated margins
- Typical location (parasagittal, transverse sinus)

Pathology
General
- Etiology-Pathogenesis
  - ○ Direct blow to skull

Skull Fracture (Fx)

- Epidemiology
  - Fx present in majority of severe head injury cases
  - 25%-35% of severely injured patients do not have skull fx
  - Skull fx absent in 25% of fatal injuries at autopsy!

Gross Pathologic or Surgical Features
- Types: Linear, depressed, diastatic
- Associated injuries
  - Linear fx: Extra-axial hematoma
  - Depressed fx: Lacerated dura, arachnoid; parenchymal injury
  - Skull base fx: Cranial nerve injury, CSF leak, epistaxis, periorbital bruising
  - 10%-15% of patients with severe head trauma (GCS 3-6) have C1 or C2 fracture

Clinical Issues
Presentation
- Varies with underlying injury

Natural History
- Varies with underlying injury
- Patients who return to ED have a remarkable incidence of missed intracranial lesions, poor outcome

Selected References
1. Hofman PAM et al: Value of radiological diagnosis of skull fracture in the management of mild head injury. J Neurol Neurosurg Psychiatr 68: 416-22, 2000
2. Vilks GM et al: Use of a complete neurological examination to screen for significant intracranial abnormalities in minor head injury. Am J Emerg Med 18: 159-63, 2000
3. Kleinman PK et al: Soft tissue swelling and acute skull fractures. J Pediatr 121: 737-9, 1992

Axonal Injury

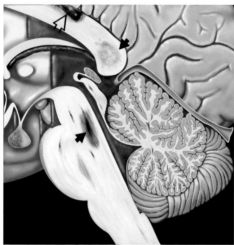

Mid-sagittal graphic depicts hemorrhagic (midbrain) and nonhemorrhagic (CC splenium) axonal injury (black arrows), traumatic IVH, SAH, and dorsolateral CC contusion (open arrow).

Key Facts
- Diffuse axonal injury (DAI) = second most common traumatic brain injury (TBI)
- **Not** caused by mechanical "shearing"
- Impaired axoplasmic transport, axonal swelling, disconnection
- Most DAI lesions are microscopic, nonhemorrhagic
- MR >> CT for detection

Imaging Findings
General Features
- Multiple lesions in nearly all cases
- Best diagnostic sign = hemorrhages at gray/white matter, corpus callosum, fornix, upper brainstem, basal ganglia, internal capsule
CT Findings
- May be normal, especially with mild TBI
- 20%-50% demonstrate petechial hemorrhage(s)
- 10%-20% evolve to focal mass lesion
MR Findings
- Multiple high-signal foci on T2WI, FLAIR
- Low signal on T2* sequences
Other Modality Findings
- Decreased ADC
- MRS: Decreased NAA/Cr correlates with outcome
- MSI: Abnormal low-frequency magnetic activity
Imaging Recommendations
- Follow-up at 24h (1/6 evolve)

Differential Diagnosis
Nonhemorrhagic DAI
- Multifocal white matter hyperintensities on T2WI
  - Demyelinating disease (ovoid, may enhance)

Axonal Injury

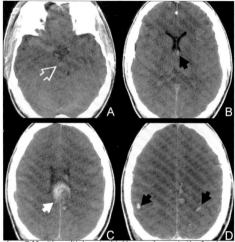

NECT scans show DAI with multiple petechial hemorrhages in the fornix and subcortical WM (black arrows), dorsolateral CC contusion (white arrow), and tSAH (open arrow).

- o Small vessel disease, lacunar infarcts (older patients)
- o Metastases (enhance)

Hemorrhagic DAI
- Multiple "black dots" on T2-, T2*
  - o Hypertensive microhemorrhages (longstanding chronic HTN)
  - o Amyloid angiopathy (elderly, normotensive, often demented)
  - o Cavernous/capillary malformations (mixed hemorrhages)

Pathology
General
- Etiology-Pathogenesis
  - o Inertial forces in nonimpact injuries
  - o Rapid head rotation
  - o Differential acceleration/deceleration
  - o Axons rarely disconnected or "sheared" (only in most severe injury)
  - o Non-disruptively injured axons undergo
    - Traumatic depolarization
    - Massive ion fluxes, spreading depression
    - Excitatory amino acid release
    - Metabolic alterations
    - Cellular swelling
    - Accelerated glycolysis, lactate accumulation
  - o Result
    - Secondary "axotomy"
    - Impaired axoplasmic transport
    - Disconnection
    - Wallerian degeneration, diffuse deafferention
- Epidemiology
  - o Second most common lesion in CHI
  - o Occurs in slightly less than 50% of cases

o   80%-100% autopsy prevalence in fatal injuries

Gross Pathologic or Surgical Features
- Multiple small round/ovoid/linear white matter lesions
- Widely distributed
  o   Parasagittal white matter
  o   Corpus callosum
  o   Brain stem tracts (e.g., medial lemnisci, corticospinal tracts)

Microscopic Features
- Axonal swellings, "retraction" balls
- Microglial clusters
- Macro-, microhemorrhages (torn penetrating vessels)

Clinical Issues

Presentation
- Immediate coma typical
- Brainstem damage (pontomedullary rent) associated with immediate or early death
- Mild DAI can occur without coma

Natural History
- Variable course
- Post-concussion syndrome (persistent HA, cognitive decline, personality changes)

Treatment & Prognosis
- Variable: TBI = 80% mild, 10% moderate, 10% severe
- Admission GCS does not always correlate with outcome
- In absence of expanding mass lesion (e.g., EDH) DAI is commonest cause of post-traumatic coma, vegetative state
- Significant genomic responses to brain trauma occur
  o   Induction of "immediate early genes"
  o   Activation of multiple signal transduction pathways
  o   Apolipoprotein E (apoE) genotype, amyloid deposition may influence clinical outcome

Selected References
1.   Sinson G et al: MTI and proton MRS in the evaluation of axonal injury. AJNR 22: 143-51, 2001
2.   Kuzma BB, Goodman JM: Improved identification of axonal shear injuries with gradient echo MR technique. Surg Neurol 53: 400-2, 2000
3.   Graham DI et al: Neurotrauma. Brain Pathol 7: 1285-8, 1997

Cortical Contusions

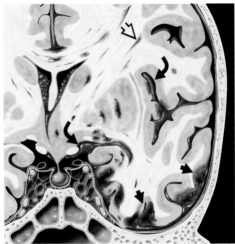

Coronal graphic depicts cortical contusions (black arrows), DAI (open arrow), and traumatic SAH (curved arrows).

Key Facts
- Most common parenchymal injury
- Gyri impact bone
- Imaging findings worsen with time

Imaging Findings

General Features
- Best diagnostic sign = patchy superficial hemorrhages, edema
- Most common sites
    - Anteroinferior temporal lobes
    - Perisylvian cortex
    - Anteroinferior frontal lobes
- Less common
    - Parasagittal ("gliding" contusions)
    - Dorsal corpus callosum
    - Dorsolateral brainstem (perimesencephalic SAH common)

CT Findings
- May be normal early
- Evolve with time (1/6 cases develop focal mass)
- Low-density cortex mixed with multifocal high-density lesions (petechial hemorrhages)
- Subacute contusions may enhance
- Associated lesions
    - Skull fracture 35%
    - Soft-tissue (scalp, subgaleal) contusions 70%
    - SDH, traumatic SAH, IVH common
- Secondary lesions (e.g., herniations, perfusion disturbances) common

MR Findings
- MR > CT in detecting presence, delineating extent of lesions
- Acute contusions

Cortical Contusions

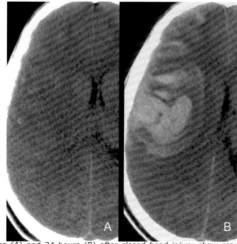

NECT scans (A) and 24 hours (B) after closed head injury show marked interval worsening of cortical contusions.

- o   Multifocal mixed signal lesions
  - ▪ Edematous cortex hyperintense on T2WI, FLAIR
  - ▪ Acute hemorrhage isointense on T1-, hypo- on T2WI
  - ▪ Hemorrhage "blooms" on T2* sequences
- • Subacute
  - o   Mixed hypo-, hyperintense
- • Chronic
  - o   Edema, mass effect subside
  - o   Focal/diffuse parenchymal atrophy
  - o   Hemosiderin, ferritin deposits
    - ▪ Hypointense on T2WI
    - ▪ "Bloom" on T2*
    - ▪ 10% show no hemosiderin on standard spin-echo scans

Differential Diagnosis
- • None

Pathology
General
- • Etiology-Pathogenesis
  - o   Injury occurs at initial impact
  - o   Gyral crests contact bone (less often dura)
- • Epidemiology
  - o   Most common parenchymal lesion in head trauma
  - o   Present in nearly half of moderate/severe CHI cases
  - o   Multiple, bilateral lesions in 90%
Gross Pathologic or Surgical Features
- • Contusions
  - o   "Coup" = lesion(s) with main acceleration blow
  - o   "Contrecoup" = lesion(s) opposite impact site

Cortical Contusions

- ○ Often evolve
  - ▪ Petechial hemorrhages, edema form along gyral crests
  - ▪ Small hemorrhages may coalesce, worsen
  - ▪ Large hematomas may occur as early as 30-60 mins
  - ▪ Delayed hematomas may develop 24-48h later
- Lacerations
  - ○ Intracerebral hematoma with "burst" lobe
  - ○ aSDH common, communicates with parenchymal hematoma through lacerated brain, torn pia-arachnoid
  - ○ tSAH common

Clinical Issues
Presentation
- Loss of consciousness less common than with DAI
- Focal neurologic deficits vary
Natural History
- Varies with extent of primary injury, associated/secondary lesions (mass effect, herniations, perfusion alterations)
- Patients who survive to have at least one admission CT scan
  - ○ Contusions more evident after 24h
  - ○ Almost 25% of patients develop diffuse brain swelling
  - ○ 20% develop new focal hematomas
Treatment & Prognosis
- +/- Evacuate focal hematoma
- Mitigate secondary effects of CHI
  - ○ Raised intracranial pressure
  - ○ Perfusion disturbances

Selected References
1. Besenski N et al: The course of the traumatising force in acceleration head injury: CT evidence. Neuroradiol 38: S36-41, 1996
2. Graham DI et al: The nature, distribution and causes of traumatic brain injury. Brain Pathol 5: 397-406, 1995
3. Gentry L: Imaging of closed head injury. Radiol 191: 1-17, 1994

Epidural Hematoma (EDH)

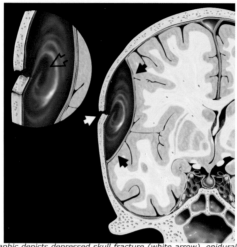

Coronal graphic depicts depressed skull fracture (white arrow), epidural hematoma (black arrows point to displaced dura). Insert shows "swirl sign" (open arrow) indicating rapid bleeding.

Key Facts
- Uncommon, potentially fatal
- Prompt recognition, appropriate treatment essential
- Classic "lucid interval" in <50%
- Hypoattenuating area ("swirl sign") = acute bleeding
- 10%-25% show delayed enlargement

Imaging Findings
General Features
- Best diagnostic sign = hyperdense biconvex extra-axial mass
- Underlying brain, subarachnoid space compressed
- Gray-white interface displaced
- Herniation common

CT Findings
- Skull fracture in 85%-90%
- Nearly all EDHs occur at impact ("coup") site
- 2/3 hyperdense; 1/3 mixed hyper/hypo
  - Low density "swirl sign" = active bleeding
  - Gas bubbles up to 20%
- 1/3-1/2 have other significant lesions
  - "Contrecoup" SDH
  - Contusions
- Secondary effects common
  - Perfusion alterations
  - Herniations (subfalcine, descending transtentorial)

MR Findings
- Thin black line between EDH, brain = displaced dura
- Acute EDH isointense with cortex on most sequences

Other Modality Findings
- DSA
  - Avascular lentiform-shaped mass

Epidural Hematoma (EDH)

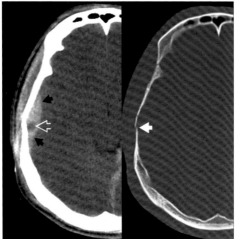

NECT scans show slightly depressed skull fracture (white arrow), hyperdense EDH (black arrows) with a hypodense swirl sign (open arrow).

- ○ Cortical arteries displaced away from skull
- ○ May displace dural venous sinus
- ○ Middle meningeal artery (MMA) laceration (rare)
  - ▪ "Tram track" sign (contrast extravasates from MMA into paired middle meningeal veins)
- MRA
  - ○ Demonstrates displaced venous sinus, if present

Differential Diagnosis
Nontraumatic Hyperdense Extraaxial Masses
- Meningioma (enhances)
- Metastasis (adjacent skull lesion common)
- Dural tuberculoma (enhances)
- Extramedullary hematopoiesis (history of blood dyscrasia)

Pathology
General
- Etiology-Pathogenesis (lacerated vessel)
  - ○ 85%-90% MMA
  - ○ 10%-15% other (dural sinus)
- Epidemiology
  - ○ 1%-4% of imaged trauma patients
  - ○ 10% autopsy prevalence
Gross Pathologic or Surgical Features
- Hematoma collects between calvarium, outer dura
  - ○ Temporoparietal most common site
  - ○ May cross midline, dural attachments
  - ○ Rarely crosses sutures (exception: large hematoma, diastatic fx)
- > 95% unilateral
- 90%-95% supratentorial

Epidural Hematoma (EDH)

- Uncommon
  - 5%-10% posterior fossa
  - "Vertex" EDH
    - Rare
    - Linear or diastatic fracture crosses SSS
    - Usually venous
    - Size underestimated on axial CT

Clinical Issues

Presentation
- Classic "lucid interval" in < 50%
- Signs of mass effect, herniation common
- Pupil-involving CN III palsy

Natural History
- Delayed development or enlargement common
  - 10%-25% of cases
  - Usually occurs within first 36 hours

Treatment & Prognosis
- Generally good outcome if promptly recognized, treated
  - 5% overall mortality
- Even large volume EDHs can have low morbidity
- Small EDHs sometimes followed without surgery

Selected references
1. Al-Nakshabandi NA: The swirl sign. Radiol 218: 433, 2001
2. Sullivan TP et al: Follow-up of conservatively managed epidural hematomas. AJNR 20: 107-13, 1999
3. Paterniti S et al: Is the size of an epidural hematoma related to outcome? Acta Neurochir 140: 953-5, 1998

Subdural Hematoma (SDH)

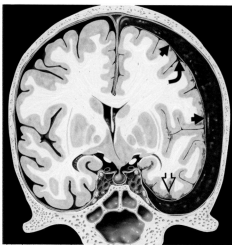

Coronal graphic depicts typical crescentic-shaped subdural hematoma (black arrows). Note cortical contusions (open arrow), subtle traumatic subarachnoid hemorrhage (curved arrow).

Key Facts
- Density decreases approximately 1.5H/day as SDH evolves
- > 70% of acute SDHs have significant associated lesions
- Use wide window settings (150-200H) to identify small SDHs

Imaging Findings
General Features
- Best diagnostic clue = "dots" of CSF in compressed sulci displaced inwards from skull
- Acute SDH (aSDH)
  - Crescentic collection over hemisphere
  - May cross sutures, not dural attachments
  - Often extends into interhemispheric fissure, along tentorium
  - Other lesions (e.g., traumatic SAH) in >70%
- Subacute SDH (sSDH)
  - Crescentic collection
- Chronic SDH (cSDH)
  - Crescentic or lentiform mass
  - Fluid hematoma + encapsulating membranes
  - Recurrent, mixed-age hemorrhages common; **in a child should raise suspicion of nonaccidental trauma!**

CT Findings
- aSDH (immediate to several days)
  - 60% high density
  - 40% mixed hyper-, hypodense (active bleed or torn arachnoid)
  - Hyperacute (unclotted) aSDH mostly hypodense
  - May be isodense if coagulopathy/anemia (Hgb < 8-10g/dl)
- sSDH (2 days-2 weeks after formation)
  - May be same density as underlying cortex
  - Gray-white junction displaced medially
  - "Dots" of CSF in compressed sulci under SDH

13

Subdural Hematoma (SDH)

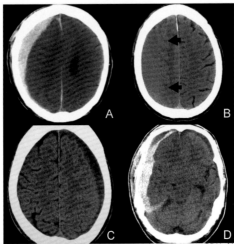

Series of NECT scans in 4 different patients depicts acute SDH (A), subacute ("isodense") SDH with displaced GW junction (B, arrows), chronic SDH (C) and chronic SDH with acute bleed (D).

- o   IV contrast may enhance displaced veins
- • cSDH (weeks-months after formation) can be classified by internal architecture/extension
  - o   Homogeneous
    - ▪ Homogeneous density
    - ▪ Can be laminar (thin, high-density layer of fresh blood along inner membrane)
  - o   Separated
    - ▪ Two layered components (high-density bottom, low-density top)
    - ▪ Sometimes density gradually changes ("gradated")
  - o   Trabecular
    - ▪ Inhomogeneous with high-density septa
    - ▪ Contents low to isodense
    - ▪ Thickened or calcified capsule
  - o   Other findings of cSDH
    - ▪ IV contrast delineates encapsulating membranes
    - ▪ +/- "Hygroma" (subdural CSF, arachnoid tear)
    - ▪ 1%-2% calcify

<u>MR Findings</u>
- • Signal varies with hematoma age
- • cSDH
  - o   Membranes enhance
  - o   Delayed scans show contrast diffusion into SDH

Differential Diagnosis
<u>cSDH</u>
- • Subdural hygroma (clear CSF, no encapsulating membranes)
- • Subdural effusion (xanthochromic fluid from extravasation of plasma from outer membrane; 20% evolve into cSDH)

Subdural Hematoma (SDH)

- Pachymeningopathies (thickened dura)
  - Chronic meningitis (may be indistinguishable)
  - Post-surgical (shunt, etc)
  - Intracranial hypotension ("slumping" midbrain, tonsillar herniation)
  - Sarcoid (nodular, "lumpy-bumpy")
  - Metastases (skull often involved)

Pathology
General
- Etiology-Pathogenesis
  - aSDH
    - Both nonimpact as well as direct injury
    - Sudden tangential, rotational acceleration
    - Cortical arteries may be torn
    - Parasagittal bridging veins disrupted
    - Blood collects between inner dural layer, arachnoid
  - sSDH
    - RBCs lyse, Hgb evolves
    - Density decreases an average of 1.5H/day
  - cSDH
    - Develops over 2-3 weeks
    - Serosanguinous fluid
    - Encapsulated by granulation tissue
    - "Neomembranes" with fragile capillaries
    - Cycle of recurrent bleeding-coagulation-fibrinolysis
    - 5% multiloculated with fluid-blood density levels
    - May continue to enlarge
- Epidemiology
  - SDHs found in 10%-20% of imaged, 30% of autopsy cases

Clinical Issues
Presentation
- Loss of consciousness; other symptoms due to focal mass lesion/diffuse brain injury

Treatment & Prognosis
- Prognosis in aSDH poor (50%-80% mortality)
  - Emergency preoperative high dose mannitol may improve outcome
- Hematoma thickness, midline shift > 20mm correlate with poor outcome
- Lethal if hematoma volume > 8-10% of intracranial volume
- Recurrence risk of cSDH varies with type ("separated" is highest; thickened or calcified membrane almost never re-hemorrhages)

Selected References
1. Nakaguchi H et al: Factors in the natural history of chronic subdural hematomas that influence their postoperative recurrence. J Neurosug 95: 256-62, 2001
2. Mori K et al: Delayed magnetic resonance imaging with Gd-DTPF differentiates subdural hygroma and subdural effusion. Surg Neurol 53: 303-11, 2000
3. Kaminogo M et al: Characteristics of symptomatic chronic subdural haematomas on high-field MRI. Neuroradiol 41: 109-16, 1999

Traumatic Subarachnoid (tSAH)

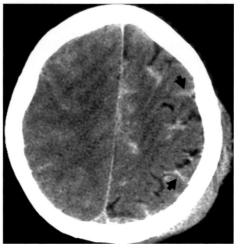

NECT scan shows edematous right hemisphere with effaced GW junction. Note traumatic SAH over left hemisphere (arrows), overlying scalp swelling.

Key Facts
- Trauma is most common cause of SAH (**not** ruptured aneurysm)!
- Amount of tSAH correlates with delayed ischemia, poor outcome

Imaging Findings
General Features
- Best diagnostic sign = high density in sulci/cisterns next to contusions or under SDH/skull fx/scalp laceration
- Looks identical to aneurysmal SAH (aSAH) except for location
  - Adjacent to contusions, SDHs
  - Convexity sulci > basal cisterns

CT Findings
- tSAH
  - High density in subarachnoid space(s)
  - Blood in interpeduncular "notch"
    - May be only manifestation of subtle SAH
- Traumatic intraventricular hemorrhage (tIVH)
  - High density in choroid plexus, ventricles
  - Blood-CSF level common
  - Usually occurs with contusions, deep parenchymal hematomas
- Intracerebral hematomas
  - Subcortical gray matter (basal ganglia), brainstem
  - Size varies from a few millimeters to several centimeters

MR Findings
- tSAH
  - Isointense with brain on T1WI ("dirty" CSF), T2WI
  - High signal on FLAIR
- tIVH
  - Focal hemorrhage in choroid plexus
  - +/- Blood-CSF level

Traumatic Subarachnoid (tSAH)

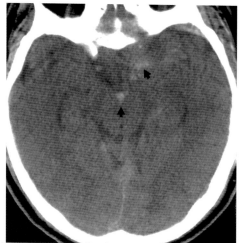

NECT scan in a patient with closed head injury shows subtle SAH in the interpeduncular fossa, Sylvian fissure (arrows).

- o Signal varies with age of clot
- Intracerebral hematomas
  - o Mixed signal core (iso-, hypointense on T1WI) with surrounding hyperintense edema (hyperintense on T2WI)

Differential Diagnosis
Aneurysmal SAH
- Aneurysm can be identified on DSA/CTA/MRA in > 85%
- Contusions, SDH, other lesions present in nearly all cases of tSAH

Pathology
General
- Etiology-Pathogenesis
  - o tSAH usually associated with contusions, SDH; probably arises from tearing of veins in subarachnoid space
  - o tIVH probably arises from shearing of choroid arteries
  - o Intracerebral hematomas arise from shearing of penetrating arteries
- Epidemiology
  - o tSAH
    - 33% with moderate brain injury; nearly 100% at autopsy
    - tSAH-associated vasospasm 2%-41% of cases
  - o tIVH
    - Uncommon
    - Reflects severity of overall trauma
    - Usually occurs with other injuries (i.e., deep hematomas)
    - Isolated tIVH occurs in 5% of cases
  - o Intracerebral hematomas
    - 2%-16% prevalence in CHI
    - May show delayed enlargement

Traumatic Subarachnoid (tSAH)

Gross Pathologic or Surgical Features
- tSAH: Acute blood over temporal lobes, in convexity sulci
- tIVH: Blood-CSF levels in ventricles
- Intracerebral hematomas: Blood interspersed with contused, edematous brain

Clinical Issues
Presentation
- Depends on associated injuries

Natural History
- tSAH
  - Acute hydrocephalus rare
  - Vasospasm
    - May develop quickly (2-3 days post-injury)
    - Peaks 2 weeks after injury
    - Uncommon cause of post traumatic infarct
- tIVH: Gradually clears
- Intracerebral hematomas: Often coalesce, enlarge

Treatment and Prognosis
- tSAH
  - Presence on initial CT scan correlates with poor outcome
  - May improve with therapy
- tIVH
  - Rarely may develop intra- or extraventricular obstructive hydrocephalus

Selected References
1. Server A et al: Post-traumatic cerebral infarction. Acta Radiol 42: 254-60, 2001
2. Boto GR et al: Basal ganglia hematomas in severely head injured patients. J Neurosurg 94: 224-32, 2001
3. Gentry LR: Imaging of closed head injury. Radiol 191: 1-17, 1994

Non-Accidental Trauma (N.A.T.)

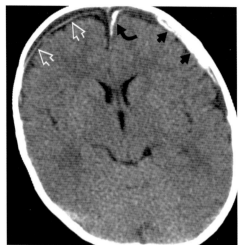

NECT scan shows layered hyper/hypodense SDHs on the left (black arrows) and a definite subdural membrane on the right (open white arrows). Note interhemispheric extension of aSDH (curved arrow). Non-accidental trauma.

Key Facts
- N.A.T. = most common cause of traumatic death in infancy
- Cause of death usually brain swelling (not hemorrhage)
- Infants have relatively large head, weak neck muscles
- Shaking/impact => torn bridging veins, retinal schisis
- Upper cervical cord stretching => apnea => ischemic brain injury

Imaging Findings
General Features
- Best diagnostic sign = infant/young child with multiple hemorrhages, different ages

CT Findings
- Acute SDH along tentorium, interhemispheric fissure
- tSAH/convexity "smears" of blood
- Focal or diffuse edema
- Subdural hygroma/cSDH, atrophy in 30% - 45%

MR Findings
- Mixed signal intensity SDHs (acute superimposed on chronic)
- Slit-like tears in subcortical white matter
- Sequelae: Global atrophy, delayed myelination

Other Modality Findings
- Skull film: Fracture type, specificity for N.A.T.
  - Linear (low)
  - Compound (moderate)
  - Fractures crossing midline/sutures (high)
- Skeletal survey
  - Skeleton = most common site of inflicted injury
  - Healing fractures of differing ages!
  - Metaphyseal corner fractures
  - (Posterior) rib fractures; scapular, sternal fractures

Non-Accidental Trauma (N.A.T.)

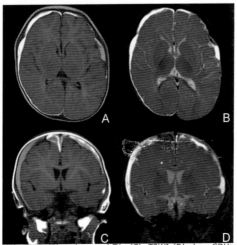

Axial FLAIR (A), T2WI (B) and coronal T1- (C), T2WI (D) show SDHs of different signal intensities, ages. N.A.T.

- T-L compression fxs, spinous process avulsion fractures
- Abdominal CT: Solid visceral injury (common > 1y)
- DWI
  - Acute
    - Increased conspicuity of abnormalities in unmyelinated brain
    - Shows restricted diffusion (high signal)
  - Chronic
    - DWI/FLAIR "mismatch" (DWI no restriction, FLAIR high-signal areas) may confirm multiple episodes of brain injury
- MRS: Shows ↓NAA, ↑Ch/Cr ratio, ↑lactate/lipid peaks

Imaging Recommendations
- NECT +/- MR to document hemorrhage age, sequelae
- Skeletal survey +/- scintigraphy (if > 2y or if skeletal survey equivocal, clinical suspicion high)
- Abdominal CT if multiple injuries, abnormal LFT, or coma

Differential Diagnosis
Accidental Trauma
- Appropriate history for degree of injury

Uncommon
- Brain: Coagulopathies (hemophilia, leukemia)
- Skeletal abnormalities: Osteogenesis imperfecta, rickets, syphilis
- Metabolic: Glutaric acidura type 1, Menkes

Pathology
General
- General (autopsy)
  - 85% signs of head impact (skull fx/subscalp bruising)
  - 50% significant extracranial injuries

Non-Accidental Trauma (N.A.T.)

- Etiology-Pathogenesis-Pathophysiology
  - Mechanism: Shaking/direct impact, rotational/angular deceleration, acceleration/deceleration (whiplash)
  - Reason infants are vulnerable: Large head:body ratio + weak neck muscles, developing brain
  - **Minor falls do not typically cause the requisite rotational forces needed for spectrum of brain injuries seen in N.A.T.!!**
- Epidemiology
  - Risk factors
    - <1y, prematurity, twin
    - Male, stepchild
    - Physical handicap
    - Low socioeconomic status
    - Young parents

Gross Pathology
- Diffuse brain swelling (cause of death in 80%)
- aSDH 72% (larger volume SDHs in older children)
- 20% evidence for prior brain injury (cSDH, etc)
- tSAH 50% (often co-exists with fracture and/or SDH)
- Retinal hemorrhage 70%-80% (usually bilateral, always with SDH)
- Skull fractures 36% (majority parietooccipital)
- Healing fxs of differing ages
- EDH very rare in N.A.T.

Microscopic Features
- Severe HIE 78%
- Cortical contusions, lacerations < 10%
- Classical DAI only 6%

Clinical Issues

Presentation
- **Discordance between stated HX, injury on imaging!** (history of minimal or no trauma)
- Poor feeding, vomiting, irritability, seizures, lethargy, coma, apnea

Natural History & Prognosis
- High mortality 15-38% (60% if coma at initial presentation)
- Almost 50% of survivors have neurologic deficits
- Factors associated with poor outcome
  - Clinical: Low admission GCS, need for intubation, prolonged coma, poor visual/pupillary response, age <6 months
  - Imaging: Edema/ischemia, abnormal MRS

Treatment
- Notification to local Child Protection Agency mandated in US /Canada / Australia /some European countries
- Multidisciplinary child abuse and neglect team intervention (to prevent further injury to child/siblings)

Selected References
1. Geddes et al: Neuropathology of inflicted head injury in children: 1. Patterns of brain damage. 2. Microscopic brain injury in infants. Brain 124(Pt 7): 1290-1306, 2001
2. Ewing-Cobbs et al: Acute neuroradiologic findings in young children with inflicted or noninflicted traumatic brain injury. Child's Nerv System 16; 25-34, 2000
3. Duhaime A-C et al: Nonaccidental head injury in infants- the "Shaken-baby syndrome". NEJM 338:1822-9, 1998

Cerebral Edema

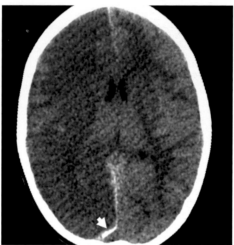

NECT scan in a child with nonaccidental trauma shows edematous right hemisphere with loss of GM-WM interfaces. A small interhemispheric SDH is present (arrow).

Key Facts
- Brain/CSF/blood exist in closed intracranial compartment
- To maintain normal ICP, increase in one must be balanced by decrease in others (Monro-Kellie)
- Two basic forms of brain edema, vasogenic and cytotoxic
- Both have astrocytic swelling, often co-exist
- Cerebral edema is important secondary effect of trauma, ischemia

Imaging Findings
General Features
- Best diagnostic sign = focal/diffuse increase in brain water
- Biphasic pattern in trauma
  - Immediate vasogenic edema
  - Cytotoxic edema within hours
  - Usually adjacent to/mixed with contused brain
  - Can be diffuse
    - Older children/adolescents
    - May follow sustained posttraumatic cerebral hypoperfusion in immature brain
- Post-traumatic edema generally resolves within 2 weeks
- Atrophy ensues

CT Findings
- NECT
  - Low-density brain substance, WM > GM
    - Subcortical WM less resistant to fluid accumulation than GM
    - Loss of GM/WM interfaces
  - In CHI, often mixed with high density (hemorrhage)
  - Compressed ventricles/effaced sulci
  - Vasogenic more prominent in WM, cytotoxic more prominent in GM

Cerebral Edema

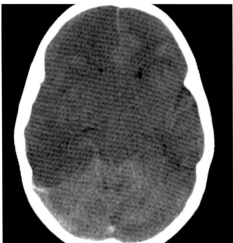

Follow-up scan 24h later shows diffuse low density in both hemispheres with "white cerebellum" sign. Brain death was documented on isotope flow study.

- o Decreased supratentorial perfusion with preservation of infratentorial perfusion => "white cerebellum" sign
- CECT
  - o Usually no enhancement unless BBB disrupted

<u>MR Findings</u>
- Hypo- on T1-, hyperintense on T2WI
- Patchy enhancement if BBB breakdown

<u>Other Modality Findings</u>
- DWI
  - o Vasogenic: Increased brain water (increased ADC)
  - o Cytotoxic: Cellular swelling (decreased ADC)
- MRS: Decreased NAA, elevated Cho (membrane breakdown)
- PET/SPECT: Show decreased rCBV, hypometabolism
- MRA: May show decreased flow/brain perfusion

Differential Diagnosis
<u>Anoxic Encephalopathy</u>
<u>Metabolic Encephalopathy</u>
- Uremia
- Hypertensive encephalopathy
- Elevated venous pressure
- Mitochondrial disorders (e.g., MELAS)

Pathology
<u>General</u>
- General Path Comments
  - o Increased brain water
  - o Astroglial swelling (not reactive astrogliosis)
- Etiology-Pathogenesis-Pathophysiology
  - o Vasogenic edema
    - BBB breakdown

- Endothelial tight junctions disrupted => leakage of proteins/Na++/water => pressure-driven fluid influx in extracellular spaces
- Primarily WM, myelin (major association bundles, relative sparing of commissural/projection fibers)
  - ○ Cytotoxic edema
    - Intracellular (closed barrier) edema
    - Energy failure => loss of Na++/K homeostasis
    - Intracellular water uptake causes cell swelling, contraction of extracellular space
  - ○ Other brain water disturbances
    - Hydrocephalic (interstitial) = increased intraventricular volume/pressure drives CSF through ventricular lining
    - Hydrostatic (congestive)= high intravascular pressure => cerebrovascular resistance increase=> flooding capillary beds
    - Hypoosmotic = flooding with IV fluids, inappropriate secretion of antidiuretic hormone, multiple, bilateral lesions in 90%

Gross Pathologic or Surgical Features
- Increased brain water, obliteration of cisterns/ventricles/sulci

Microscopic Features
- Changes related to hypoxemia and brain death

Clinical Issues
Presentation
- Varies with primary injury

Natural History
- Slowly expanding lesions can be accommodated without elevated ICP
- Rapid expansion (trauma, rapid tumor growth, abscess)
  - ○ Rapid rise of ICP
  - ○ "Cascade" of sequelae (e.g., excitotoxin release)
  - ○ Cell death

Treatment & Prognosis
- Goal = maintain cerebral perfusion pressure without inducing hydrostatic vasogenic edema
- Osmotherapy/neuroprotective agents/steroids controversial

Selected References
1. Bauer R et al: Ontogenetic aspects of traumatic brain edema – facts and suggestions. Exp Toxicol Pathol 51: 143-50, 1999
2. Pollay M. Blood-brain barrier; Cerebral edema. In Wilkins RH, Rengachary SS (eds), Neurosurgery, 2nd ed, McGraw-Hill, 1996
3. Barzo P et al: MRI diffusion-weighted spectroscopy of reversible and irreversible ischemic injury following closed head injury. Acta Neurochir Suppl (Wien) 70:115-18, 1997

Vascular Effects of Trauma

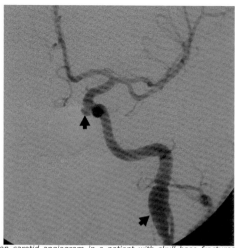

Left common carotid angiogram in a patient with skull base fractures shows two traumatic pseudoaneurysms (arrows).

Key Facts
- Hemodynamic alterations (local, regional, general perfusion disturbances) common with TBI
- Pseudoaneurysm, dissection, vessel laceration, AVF less common vascular causes of delayed clinical deterioration
- Vascular lesions from penetrating head trauma differ in pathogenesis and clinical sequelae from nonpenetrating injuries

Imaging Findings
General Features
- Vasospasm, laceration, dissection, pseudoaneurysm, focal and generalized hypoperfusion, frank cerebral infarcts may all occur
- >80% of cervical vascular injuries involve carotid arteries

CT Findings
- NECT (vary with lesion)
  - Focal hematoma (pseudoaneurysm)
  - Cortical/white matter hypodensities
    - Ischemia (vasospasm, embolic infarcts)
  - Secondary infarcts from brain herniation
    - DTH: PCA occlusion
    - Subfalcine: ACA occlusion
    - Central: Basal perforating vessel occlusions
  - Dilated arteries, veins/dural sinus (traumatic AVF)

MR Findings
- Acute hematoma (usually iso- on T1, hypointense on T2WI)
- Ischemia: Hypointense foci on T1WI, hyperintense on T2WI, FLAIR

Other Modality Findings
- DSA (penetrating neck injury)
  - Most common carotid injury = occlusion (35%)
  - Pseudoaneurysm (33%)
  - Intimal flaps and dissections (33%)

Vascular Effects of Trauma

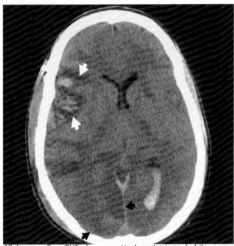

NECT scan 48 hours after CHI shows cortical contusions (white arrows) and IVH. Descending herniation resulted in PCA occlusion with occipital infarct (black arrows).

- o   AVF
- o   Vasospasm (segmental/generalized arterial narrowing)
- • DSA (traumatic intracranial aneurysm)
  - o   50% involve MCA
  - o   25% distal ACA
  - o   25% petrous/cavernous ICA or BA
- • CTA
  - o   High sensitivity, specificity in penetrating neck trauma
  - o   Single or multiple regions of intracranial hypoperfusion
  - o   Wall irregularity, caliber changes
  - o   Contrast extravasation
  - o   Lack of intravascular enhancement
- • MRA: Vessel occlusion, regional hypoperfusion
- • DWI: Restricted diffusion (high signal)
- • Transcranial Doppler (trauma-induced vasospasm)
  - o   Elevated peak MCA velocity (V_{MCA})
  - o   Increased "hemispheric ratio" ($V_{MCA}/V_{EC\text{-}ICA}$)

Differential Diagnosis
Vasospasm vs. Dissection
- • MR/MRA shows intimal flap, intra- or paravascular hematoma
Large Contusion vs. Hematoma from Traumatic Pseudoaneurysm
- • Dynamic enhanced MR/MRA or CTA shows aneurysm

Pathology
General
- • Etiology-Pathogenesis
  - o   Direct penetrating trauma (e.g., ballistic injury)
  - o   Nonpenetrating (blunt) injury

Vascular Effects of Trauma

- Vertebral artery injuries more common than carotid
  - Seen in 46% of transverse foramen fxs, 75% of facet dislocations
  - Carotid stretched with rapid deceleration, hyperextension, rotation of neck
  - Intracranial injury from basal skull fx or arterial impaction against skull/dura
  - Emboli (from intimal flap, dissection, pseudoaneurysm, etc.)
  - Indirect injury
    - Vasospasm
    - Blood-brain barrier disruption with vasogenic edema
    - Excitatory amino acids induce cellular ("cytotoxic") swelling
- Epidemiology
  - 17%-36% of patients with penetrating trauma have vascular injury
  - Low prevalence (0.67%) with blunt trauma

Clinical Issues

Presentation
- Unexplained clinical deterioration, appearance of delayed/atypical hematoma should prompt search for possible vascular injury
- Clinical examination
  - Low sensitivity (60%) for detecting vascular injury
  - Symptoms often delayed (12-24h up to several weeks)
  - Varies with type of injury
- Rare but potentially life-threatening = sphenoid sinus fx with massive epistaxis and traumatic carotid pseudoaneurysm

Treatment & Prognosis
- Monitoring for ischemia, hyperemia, vasospasm is a "must"
- Consider endovascular therapy for pseudoaneurysm, etc.

Selected References
1. Server A et al: Post-traumatic cerebral infarction. Acta Radiol 42: 254-60, 2001
2. Redekop G et al: Treatment of traumatic aneurysms and arteriovenous fistulas of the skull base by using endovascular stents. J Neurosurg 95: 412-419, 2001
3. LeBlang SD et al: Noninvasive imaging of cervical vascular injuries. AJR 174: 1269-78, 2000

Herniations

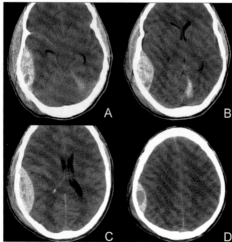

NECT scans show a rapidly developing EDH with right to left displacement (subfalcine herniation) of the lateral ventricles.

Key Facts
- Secondary effects often more devastating than primary injury
- Herniations, increased ICP, altered cerebral hemodynamics and fluid distribution exacerbate severity of initial injury

Imaging Findings
General Features
- Best diagnostic sign = displacement/effacement of CSF structures (ventricles, sulci)
- Brain, vessels shifted from one compartment into another

CT Findings
- Subfalcine herniation
  - ○ Cingulate gyrus displaced under falx
  - ○ Lateral ventricles displaced towards opposite side
  - ○ Ipsilateral ventricle compressed
  - ○ Foramen of Monro obstructs, opposite lateral ventricle enlarges
  - ○ ACA displaced, may become occluded
- Unilateral descending transtentorial herniation (DTH)
  - ○ Early
    - ▪ Uncus, parahippocampal gyrus protrude medially
    - ▪ Ipsilateral suprasellar cistern effaced
  - ○ Late
    - ▪ Suprasellar cistern completely obliterated
    - ▪ Brainstem shifts away from mass (may become compressed against tentorium, forming "Kernohan notch")
    - ▪ CN III compressed
    - ▪ PCA displaced inferomedially, may occlude (occipital infarct)
- Bilateral DTH ("central" herniation)
  - ○ Severe uni- or bilateral supratentorial mass effect
  - ○ Both hemispheres, basal nuclei pushed downwards
  - ○ Diencephalon, midbrain displaced inferiorly through incisura

Herniations

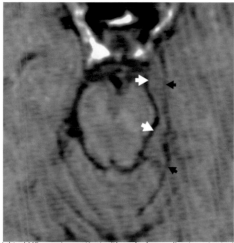

Axial T1-weighted MR scan in a patient with early descending transtentorial herniation shows the temporal lobe (white arrows) displaced medially over the tentorium (black arrows).

- o Both temporal lobes herniate into tentorial hiatus
- o Penetrating arteries often occlude, cause basal infarcts
- Ascending transtentorial herniation
  - o Vermis, cerebellum pushed up through incisura
  - o Quadrigeminal cistern deformed
  - o Midbrain displaced anteriorly
  - o May obstruct aqueduct, cause hydrocephalus
- Transalar herniation
  - o Uncommon
  - o Can be ascending (caused by large middle fossa mass) or descending (large frontal mass)
  - o Temporal lobe, MCA displaced across greater sphenoid wing
- Tonsillar herniation
  - o Tonsils pushed down, impacted into foramen magnum
  - o Cisterna magna obliterated
  - o Fourth ventricle may obstruct, cause IVOH
- Transdural/transcranial herniation
  - o Skull fx + dural laceration (may also occur with craniotomy)
  - o Elevated ICP
  - o Brain extrudes through torn dura
  - o May extend under galea

MR Findings
- DTH
  - o Findings on axial, coronal studies similar to CT
  - o Sagittal (see "Intracranial Hypotension" diagnosis)
    - ▪ Midbrain displaced inferiorly ("slumps")
    - ▪ Angle between midbrain, pons becomes more acute
    - ▪ Optic chiasm/hypothalamus displaced downwards, draped over sella
    - ▪ +/- Secondary tonsillar herniation

Herniations

- Hemodynamic effects of herniations
  - Diffuse perfusion disturbances
  - Vascular occlusion, infarcts
  - Diffuse cerebral edema, gyral swelling

Differential Diagnosis
Intracranial Hypotension Syndrome
- Dural thickening, enhancement

Pathology
General
- Etiology-Pathogenesis
  - Hemorrhage, extracellular fluid accumulate within closed space
  - CSF spaces (cisterns, ventricles) initially compressed
  - If added intracranial volume can't be accommodated
    - Gross mechanical displacement of brain, vessels occurs
    - Brain herniates
  - Exacerbates severity of primary injuries
  - May cause secondary ischemia, infarction
    - PCA occlusion, occipital infarct most common
    - ACA occlusion, distal (cingulate gyrus) infarcts
    - Perforating vessels, basal ganglia, capsule infarcts
    - Midbrain ("Duret") hemorrhage
Gross Pathologic or Surgical Features
- Grossly swollen, edematous brain
- Gyri compressed, flattened against calvarium
- Sulci effaced

Clinical Issues
Presentation
- Pupil-involving CN III palsy
- Decreased brainstem blood flow, cardiovascular collapse
- Decerebrate posturing
- Kernohan notch
  - "False localizing signs"
  - Ipsilateral hemiplegia (compression of opposite cerebral peduncle against tentorium)
Natural History
- Brain death if intracranial pressure continues to rise, mass effect progresses unabated
Treatment Issues
- Aimed at mitigating secondary effects of trauma
- Prolonged posttraumatic brain hypersensitivity
  - May offer potential "therapeutic window"
  - Possible use of neuroprotective agents

Selected References
1. Juul N et al: Intracranial hypertension and cerebral perfusion pressure. J Neurosurg 92: 1-6, 2000
2. Laine FJ et al: Acquired intracranial herniations. AJR 165: 967-73, 1995
3. Povlishock JT et al: Are the pathobiological changes evoked by traumatic brain injury immediate and irreversible? Brain Pathol 5: 415-26, 1995

Brain Death (BD)

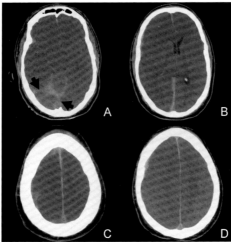

NECT scans show diffuse post-traumatic cerebral edema. Note GW effacement. Hemispheres appear low density compared to "white" cerebellum (A, arrows).

Key Facts
- BD = complete, irreversible cessation of brain function
- BD is anatomically, physiologically complex
- Legal criteria vary with jurisdiction
- BD is primarily a clinical diagnosis
- **Imaging may confirm but does not substitute for clinical criteria!**

Imaging Findings
General Features
- Best diagnostic sign = no flow in intracranial arteries/venous sinuses
- Diffuse cerebral edema
- CSF spaces compressed, gyri swollen

CT Findings
- No intravascular enhancement
- Diffuse cerebral edema
  - Loss of gray/white matter differentiation
  - "Reversal sign" (density of cerebellum >> hemispheres)
  - Low-density brain may make vessels in basal cisterns appear hyperdense, should not be mistaken for SAH!

MR Findings
- No intracranial "flow voids"
- Brain herniation (central DTH, tonsillar)
- Gyral swelling with poor gray/white differentiation
  - Cortex hyperintense on T2WI, FLAIR
- Increased enhancement of facial structures
- DWI: Diffuse hemispheric hyperintensity, severe drop in ADPC

Other Modality Findings
- DSA/MRA/CTA
  - No intracranial flow
  - Contrast stasis (ECA fills, supraclinoid ICA doesn't)

Brain Death (BD)

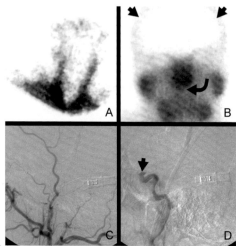

Brain death is depicted by no intracranial flow on isotope study (A). (B) "Light bulb" (arrows) and "hot nose" (curved arrow) signs. (C, D) Common carotid angiogram shows contrast stasis in ICA, no intracranial blood flow (D, arrow).

- DWI
  - Diffuse hemispheric high intensity
  - Severe drop in ADC
- Radionuclide (perfusion scanning, angiography)
  - Absence of arterial flow on dynamic study
  - No significant intracranial activity
  - Normal/increased extracranial activity ("hot nose" sign)
- Orbital Doppler
  - Absence/reversal of end-diastolic flow in ophthalmic, central retinal arteries
  - Marked increase in resistive indices in intracranial arteries
- Transcranial Doppler
  - Global circulatory arrest
  - Oscillating "to and fro" signal
  - Systolic spike
  - Absent signal

Differential Diagnosis
Technical Difficulty
Missed Bolus
Catheter-Induced Vasospasm
Diffuse Cerebral Edema from Reversible Cause
Status Epilepticus
Drug Overdose

Pathology
General
- Etiology-Pathogenesis-Pathophysiology
  - Severe cell swelling elevates intracranial pressure (ICP)
  - Markedly elevated ICP decreases CBF

- o If ICP > end-diastolic pressure in cerebral arteries, diastolic reversal occurs
- o If ICP > systolic pressure, blood flow ceases
- o Complete and irreversible loss of brain function

Gross Pathologic or Surgical Features
- Markedly swollen brain with severely compressed sulci
- Central (complete bilateral descending transtentorial) herniation
  - o Downwards displacement of basal brain structures, midbrain
  - o "Grooving" of both temporal lobes by tentorial incisura

Clinical Issues
Presentation
- Profound coma (GCS = 3) "known cause"
- Profound but reversible causes of coma must be excluded!
- Clinical diagnosis of BD highly reliable if
  - o Examiners are experienced
  - o Examiners use established criteria

Natural History
- Ancillary studies (absent BAERS, "isoelectric" cortical EEG, no intracranial flow on imaging studies) help confirm clinical Dx
- Brain stem death ensues
  - o Absent reflexes (ocular microtremor, etc.)
  - o Apnea test

Selected References
1. Nakahara M et al: Diffusion-weighted MR and apparent diffusion coefficient in the evaluation of severe brain injury. Acta Radiol 42: 365-9, 2001
2. Flowers WMJr et al: Accuracy of clinical evaluation in the determination of brain death. So. Med. J. 93: 203-6, 2000
3. Powner DJ, et al: Current considerations in the issue of brain death. Neurosurg 45: 1222-7, 1999

INFECTION

Meningitis

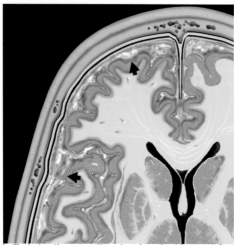

Axial graphic illustrates the serpentine pia-subarachnoid space infection (arrows) that is the most common pattern in acute pyogenic meningitis.

Key Facts
- Meningitis is a clinical-laboratory diagnosis!
- Pathology generally same regardless of agent
- Imaging findings nonspecific
- Imaging best delineates complications

Imaging Findings
General Features
- May be normal early
- Subarachnoid space, pia enhance
- Hydrocephalus often occurs as early complication
- Best diagnostic sign = positive CSF (lumbar puncture)!

CT Findings
- NECT
  - Mild ventricular enlargement
  - Basal cisterns effaced
- CECT
  - Enhancing exudate in sulci, cisterns
  - Low density areas related to perfusion alterations

MR Findings
- Exudate is isointense on T1WI, high signal on T2WI, enhances
- FLAIR shows high signal in sulci, cisterns
- Complications
  - Extraventricular obstructive hydrocephalus
  - Ventriculitis, choroid plexitis
  - Cerebrovascular (arteritis, infarction, venous thrombosis)
    - Cerebral edema, infarction
    - DWI, SPECT useful in depicting perfusion alterations

Other Modality Findings
- U/S: Sulcal enlargement, echogenic deposits in subarachnoid space
- DSA/MRA/CTA: Arterial narrowing, occlusion

Meningitis

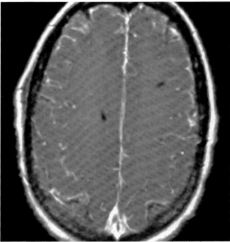

Contrast-enhanced T1WI in a patient with pyogenic meningitis demonstrates diffuse pia-subarachnoid space enhancement

Differential Diagnosis
Nonpyogenic Meningitis (e.g., Subarachnoid Metastases)
Sarcoidosis
Gadolinium in CSF
- Dialysis-dependent patient with end-stage renal disease
- Increased CSF signal on T1WI, FLAIR

Pathology
General Pathology Findings
- CNS changes grossly similar regardless of micro-organism
- Bacteria multiply in CSF
- Routes of entry to CNS
  - Hematogenous
  - Choroid plexus
- Purulent exudate fills subarachnoid space
- Pia easily penetrated by inflammatory cells, BBB altered
- Meningitis-associated brain injury
  - Cytokines
  - Reactive nitrogen species
  - Hippocampal apoptosis (cell death)
Gross Pathologic or Surgical Features
- Cisterns, sulci filled with cloudy CSF, then creamy pus
- Pia congested, may mimic SAH
- Cortex may be edematous
- Ependymitis/ventriculitis
Microscopic Features
- Meningeal exudate
  - Polymorphs
  - Fibrin
  - Intra- and extracellular bacteria

- Vessels within exudate may show fibrinoid necrosis, thrombosis
- Foci of cortical necrosis
- Infection may extend into perivascular spaces
- Subpial microglial, astrocytic proliferation

Clinical Issues
Presentation
- Malaise, fever, H/A
- Meningismus
- +/- Disturbances in mental status

Natural History
- Effective antimicrobial agents have reduced but not eliminated mortality, morbidity
- Impaired CSF resorption may cause EVOH
- Elevated ICP, cerebral perfusion alterations may occur as early complications
- Cerebritis, abscess may ensue

Selected References
1. Rai At, Hogg JP: Persistence of gadolinium in CSF: A diagnostic pitfall in patients with end-stage renal disease. AJNR 22: 1357-61, 2001
2. Andreula CF et al: CNS infections. Eur Radiol 9 (suppl 2): 15-26, 1999
3. Gray F: Bacterial infections. Brain Pathol 7: 629-47, 1997

Empyema

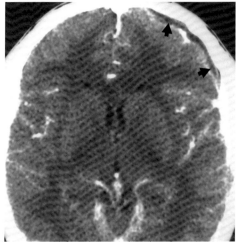

CECT scan in a patient with frontal sinusitis (not shown), meningitis, and a small left frontal subdural empyema (SDE) (arrows).

Key Facts
- Epi-, subdural empyemas (EDE, SDE) are rare, yet highly lethal
- May progress rapidly, are considered neurosurgical emergencies
- Clinical diagnosis often delayed, confused with meningitis
- MR > CT in demonstrating presence, nature, extent, complications

Imaging Findings
General Features
- Best diagnostic sign= extra-axial collection with rim enhancement
- > Two-thirds associated with sinusitis
- 15% of cases have both EDE, SDE

CT Findings
- SDE (N.B.: Can be small, easily overlooked!)
  - Crescentic iso/hyperdense extra-axial collection
    - Convexity in >50%
    - Parafalcine in 20%
  - Strong peripheral rim enhancement
  - Sinusitis in 67%, mastoiditis in 10%
- EDE
  - Biconvex low-density collection between dura, calvarium
  - Usually adjacent to frontal sinus
  - Subgaleal abscess ("Pott's puffy tumor") common

MR Findings
- SDE
  - Signal intensity > CSF on most sequences
  - Encapsulating membranes
    - Enhance strongly
    - May be loculated, show internal fibrous strands
  - Underlying brain may be hyperintense on T2WI, FLAIR

Empyema

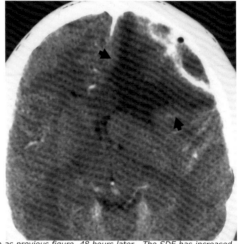

Same case as previous figure, 48 hours later. The SDE has increased. Diffuse low density in left frontal lobe (arrows) is secondary to venous infarction.

- EDE
  - Lens-shaped bifrontal or convexity collection
    - Inwardly displaced dura seen as hypointense line
  - May cross midline in frontal region
  - Posterior fossa EDE
    - Typically at sinodural angle
    - Tegmen tympani eroded
    - Pus may extend into cerebellopontine angle

Other Modality Findings
- Ultrasound
  - Useful in infants
  - Echogenic convexity collection
    - Heterogeneous
    - Hyperechoic fibrous strands
    - Thick hyperechoic inner membrane
- DWI: Restricted diffusion (increased signal intensity)

Differential Diagnosis
Chronic Subdural Hematoma
- MR shows blood products
Subdural Hygroma
- Nonenhancing CSF collection, often trauma hx
Subdural Effusion
- Sterile, nonenhancing, CSF-like collection
- Occurs in 40%-60% of infants with pyogenic meningitis

Pathology
General
- Etiology-Pathogenesis
  - Infants, young children
    - Meningitis

- ○ Older children, adults
    - ▪ Sinusitis in > 2/3
    - ▪ Direct spread through posterior wall of frontal sinus
    - ▪ Retrograde spread through valveless interconnecting venous systems of extra-, intracranial spaces
    - ▪ Mastoiditis 20%
    - ▪ Penetrating trauma (rare)
- ○ Causative organism: Streptococci, H. influenzae, S. Aureus, S. epidermidis most common

Gross Pathologic or Surgical Features
- Encapsulated, yellowish, purulent collection
- Spreads widely
    - ○ May be loculated
- Osteitis in 35%

Clinical Issues
Presentation
- Majority have fever, headaches
- Meningismus common, may mimic meningitis
- Subgaleal abscess in 1/3
- +/- Periorbital swelling
- Sinus or ear infection in > 75% of cases

Natural History
- Rapidly evolving, fulminant course
- Can be fatal unless recognized, treated
    - ○ Imaging essential as lumbar puncture can be fatal
    - ○ CSF can be normal
- Complications common
    - ○ Brain abscess 5%
    - ○ Cortical vein thrombophlebitis
    - ○ Venous ischemia
    - ○ Cerebral edema
    - ○ Hydrocephalus (> 75% of infratentorial SDEs)

Treatment & Prognosis
- Surgical drainage through wide craniotomy
- Antibiotics

Selected References
1. Nathoo N et al: Craniotomy improves outcomes for cranial subdural empyemas: Computed tomography-era experience with 699 patients. Neurosurg Oct 2001 (in press)
2. Nathoo N et al: Cranial extradural empyema in the era of computed tomography. Neurosurg 44: 754-84, 1999
3. Chen C-Y et al: Subdural empyema in 10 infants: US characteristics and clinical correlates. Radiol 207: 609-17, 1998

Abscess

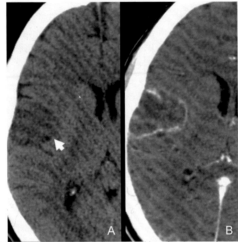

(A) NECT scan shows nonspecific right temporal low-density area (arrow). (B) CECT scan 2 days later shows poorly-delineated ring enhancement. Early cerebritis.

Key Facts
- Potentially fatal but treatable lesion
- Ring-enhancing pattern, most common finding, is also nonspecific
- DWI, MRS helpful in distinguishing abscess from mimics

Imaging Findings
<u>General Features</u>
- Best diagnostic sign= ring-enhancing lesion with high signal on DWI, low ADC
- Imaging varies with stage of abscess development
<u>CT Findings</u>
- Early cerebritis (radiological stage I)
  - May be normal early
  - Poorly-delineated hypodense subcortical lesion
  - +/- Mild patchy enhancement, mass effect
- Late cerebritis (stage II)
  - Central low density area
  - Irregular peripheral rim enhancement
  - Peripheral edema, mass effect increase
  - Gas-containing abscess rare
- Early capsule (stage III)
  - Low density center with thin, distinct enhancing capsule
    - Deepest part is thinnest; thickest near cortex
  - May be multiloculated/have "daughter" abscesses
  - Moderate vasogenic edema
- Late capsule (stage IV)
  - Cavity shrinks, capsule thickens
  - Edema, mass effect diminish
<u>MR Findings</u>
- Early cerebritis

Abscess

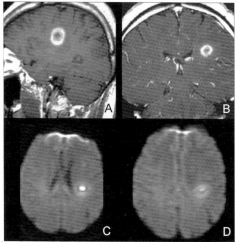

Sagittal (A) and coronal (B) enhanced T1WI show solitary ring-enhancing mass. Major DDx = abscess vs. neoplasm. (C, D) DWI shows restricted diffusion. Abscess confirmed at surgery.

- ○ T1WI: Poorly marginated, mixed hypo/hyperintense mass
- ○ T2WI: Ill-defined hyperintense mass
- ○ Patchy enhancement with contrast
- Late cerebritis
  - ○ T1WI: Hypointense center, iso-/mildly hyperintense rim
  - ○ T2WI: Hyperintense center, hypo- rim; hyperintense edema
  - ○ Intense but irregular rim enhancement
- Early capsule
  - ○ Well-defined, thin-walled enhancing rim
- Late capsule
  - ○ Cavity collapses, capsule thickens
  - ○ Edema, mass effect diminish
- Resolving abscess
  - ○ Hyperintense on T2WI, FLAIR
  - ○ Small ring/punctate enhancing focus may persist for months

<u>Other Modality Findings</u>
- DWI: Increased signal intensity
- ADC map: Markedly decreased signal
- MRS: Lactate, acetate, cytosolic amino acid resonances

Differential Diagnosis
<u>Primary or Metastatic Neoplasm</u>
- Low signal on DWI (occasionally high, can mimic abscess)
<u>Other Ring-enhancing Lesions</u>
- Resolving hematoma, MS, etc

Pathology
<u>General</u>
- Etiology-Pathogenesis

Abstract

- o Blood-borne (e.g., endocarditis, urinary tract infections)
- o Direct infection
- o Paranasal sinus, dental, otogenic infections (via valveless emissary veins)
- o Penetrating trauma (bone fragments >> metal)
- o Postoperative
- o 20%-30% have no identifiable source
  - Often polymicrobial (microaerophilic streptococci, staph)

Gross pathologic or Surgical Features
- Early cerebritis (3-5 days)
  - o Infection is focal but not localized
  - o Unencapsulated mass of PMNs, edema, scattered foci of necrosis and petechial hemorrhage
- Late cerebritis (4-5 days up to 2 weeks)
  - o Necrotic foci coalesce
  - o Rim of inflammatory cells, macrophages, granulation tissue, fibroblasts surrounds central necrotic core
  - o Vascular proliferation, surrounding vasogenic edema
- Early capsule (begins at around 2 weeks)
  - o Well-delineated collagenous capsule
  - o Liquified necrotic core, peripheral gliosis
- Late capsule (weeks to months)
  - o Central cavity shrinks
  - o Thick wall (collagen, granulation tissue, macrophages, gliosis)

Clinical Issues
Presentation
- Variable, depending on
  - o Size, location of abscess, virulence of infecting organism(s)
  - o Systemic conditions
- Headache most common symptom; fever in <50%

Natural History
- Complications of inadequately or untreated abscesses
  - o Intraventricular rupture, ventriculitis (may be fatal)
  - o Ventricular debris with irregular fluid level
  - o Hydrocephalus
  - o +/- Ependymal enhancement
  - o Meningitis, "daughter" lesions
  - o Mass effect, herniation
- Stereotactic surgery + medical Rx have greatly reduced mortality

Treatment & Prognosis
- Lumbar puncture hazardous
- Pathogen often can't be determined from CSF

Selected references
1. Tung GA et al: Diffusion-weighted MR imaging of rim-enhancing brain masses: Is markedly decreased water-diffusion specific for brain abscess? AJR 177: 709-12, 2001
2. Verlicchi A et al: From diagnostic imaging to management of brain abscesses. Riv di Neuroradiol 14: 267-74,2001
3. Fukui MB et al: CT and MR imaging features of pyogenic ventriculitis. AJNR 22: 1510-6, 2001

Encephalitis

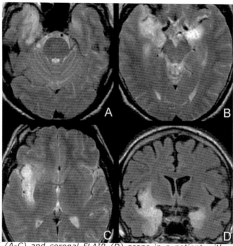

Axial T2WI (A-C) and coronal FLAIR (D) scans in a patient with early herpes encephalitis show typical cortical/subcortical high signal in both temporal lobes, right insula. FLAIR shows greater conspicuity than T2WI.

Key Facts

- Encephalitis = diffuse, nonfocal brain inflammation
- Most (but not all) caused by viruses
- Herpes = most common sporadic (nonepidemic, nonseasonal) encephalitis in temperate climates
- Can be acute (e.g., HSV) or chronic (e.g., Rasmussen encephalitis)

Imaging Findings

General Imaging Findings

- Nonspecific
- Large, poorly-delineated areas of involvement
  - Diffuse cytotoxic edema
  - +/- Patchy hemorrhage
  - +/- Meningitis
  - Minimal or no enhancement early
- Typical locations of specific acute infections
  - HSV-1 = limbic system
  - HIV-1 = cerebral white matter, brainstem; gray matter of thalamus, basal ganglia
  - Japanese encephalitis = bilateral thalami, brainstem, cerebellum
  - Enteroviral encephalomyelitis
    - EV71 (herpangina, HFMD) = posterior medulla, pons, spinal cord
    - Polio, Coxsackie = midbrain, anterior horn of spinal cord
  - Nipah viral encephalitis = multifocal white matter microinfarcts
  - St. Louis encephalitis = substantia nigra
  - Varicella-zoster virus (VZV)
    - Varicella and herpes zoster = different clinical manifestations of infection by same virus
    - <1% involve CNS

Encephalitis

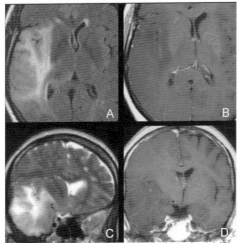

Axial FLAIR (A), coronal T2WI (C) and contrast-enhanced axial (B), coronal (D) scans in a patient with viral encephalitis show poorly-marginated, nonenhancing temporal lobe mass.

- Vasculopathy (ischemic/hemorrhagic infarctions), demyelination
- Herpes zoster oticus (Ramsay Hunt syndrome) = enhancing CNs (VII, VIII, cochlea, etc)
- Herpes zoster ophthalmicus can cause ICA necrotizing angiitis
  - Epstein-Barr virus (EBV) = symmetric basal ganglia
  - Eastern equine encephalitis = basal ganglia, thalami
  - Hantavirus = pituitary gland (hemorrhage)

CT Findings
- Initial CT negative in 75% of children with acute encephalitis
- Herpes encephalitis (HSV-1)
  - Predilection for limbic system
  - Atypical patterns seen in children
  - CT often normal early
    - Low attenuation, mild mass effect in temporal lobes, insula
    - Hemorrhage, enhancement are late features

MR Findings
- Herpes encephalitis (HSV-1)
  - Much more sensitive than CT
  - Hypo- on T1-, hyperintense on T2WI, FLAIR
  - High signal on DWI
  - +/- Mild, patchy gyriform enhancement early
  - Hemorrhage, encephalomalacia later
  - Involvement of cingulate gyrus, contralateral temporal lobe highly suggestive of herpes encephalitis
- Chronic Viral Infections
  - HIV-1 (see "HIV")
  - PML (see "HIV")

Encephalitis

- o Rasmussen encephalitis
  - Unknown agent (may be autoimmune)
  - Intractable seizures
  - Progressive hemiplegia
  - Focal cortical inflammation with tissue destruction
  - Unilateral lobar/hemisphere atrophy

Differential Diagnosis
Infiltrating Neoplasm
Ischemia
Post-infectious Syndromes

Pathology
General
- Etiology-Pathogenesis
  - o Viruses are obligate intracellular parasites
  - o Replicate in skin or mucous membranes of respiratory, GI tracts
  - o Some invade along CNs (e.g., HSV-1 via lingual nerve to trigeminal, gasserian ganglia)
  - o Latent infections may reactivate, spread along meningeal branches
  - o HSV-1 causes acute hemorrhagic, necrotizing encephalitis (primarily involving limbic system)

Clinical Issues
Presentation
- Varies widely (slight meningeal to severe encephalitic symptoms)
- +/- Fever, prodrome
- Some may cause parkinsonism
- Others (EV71, polio) may cause acute flaccid paralysis
- Segmental myoclonus suggests Nipah virus
Natural History
- Untreated, many encephalitides have high mortality, morbidity
- Rapid diagnosis, early treatment with antiviral agents can decrease mortality, may improve outcome

Selected References
1. Kleinschmidt-DeMasters BK, Gilden DH: The expanding spectrum of herpesvirus infections of the nervous system. Brain Pathol 11: 440-51, 2001
2. Theil D et al: Prevalence of HSV-1 LAT in human trigeminal, geniculate, and vestibular ganglia and its implication for cranial nerve syndromes. Brain Pathol 11: 408-13, 2001
3. Tsuchiya K et al: Diffusion-weighted MR imaging of encephalitis. AJR 173: 1097-9, 1999

HIV

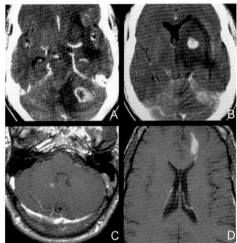

(A, B) Axial CECT scans in an HIV+ patient show ring-enhancing masses in the cerebellum, basal ganglia. Lesions regressed after anti-toxo treatment. (C, D) New lesions appeared 1 year later.

Key Facts
- Viral entry into brain occurs very early after systemic infection
- 30% of patients with AIDS have neurologic complications
- Pathology/imaging varies with patient age, acuity/chronicity
- Clinical findings should guide imaging studies (not reverse)

Imaging Findings
General Features
- Most common = white matter disease + atrophy
- Best diagnostic sign = combination of the following
  - Prominent nasopharyngeal adenoidal tissue
  - Abnormal bone marrow signal
  - Posterior triangle lymphadenopathy
  - Intraparotid cysts and/or nodes
CT Findings
- Adults: Normal/mild atrophy, white matter hypodensity
- Children: Atrophy, basal ganglia Ca++
MR Findings
- HIV encephalopathy
  - Multifocal nonenhancing white matter hyperintensities
  - Generalized atrophy
- Opportunistic infection
  - Toxoplasmosis: Ring-enhancing mass(es) basal ganglia
  - Cryptococcosis
    - Gelatinous "pseudocysts"
    - Meningoencephalitis +/- vasculitis, infarction
  - CMV-associated CNS disease
    - Encephalitis (diffuse white matter hyperintensities)
    - Ventriculitis (ependymal enhancement)

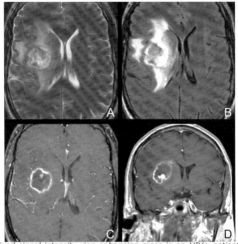

Solitary mixed signal intensity ring-enhancing mass in an HIV+ patient (A) T2WI, (B) FLAIR, (C, D) T1WI with contrast. Biopsy disclosed lymphoma.

- o Progressive multifocal leukoencephalopathy (PML)
  - ▪ White matter hyperintensities, usually don't enhance
- Lymphoma
  - o Second (to toxo) as cause of focal CNS mass in HIV+
  - o Solitary or multifocal lesions
    - ▪ Deep (basal ganglia, periventricular) > subcortical
    - ▪ Signal like gray matter (may have necrosis, hemorrhage)
    - ▪ Solid or ring-enhancing

Other Modality Findings
- DWI: Lymphoma = low signal

Imaging Recommendations (in HIV+ Patients)
- CT scan if
  - o New seizure
  - o Depressed or altered orientation
  - o Headache, different in quality (careful neurologic examination should precede neuroimaging studies)
  - o CD4 count < 200 cells/uL
- MR scan if
  - o CT shows focal mass
  - o N.B.: If routine MRI normal, contrast reveals abnormality in only 2% of cases
  - o If MR shows mass: Obtain DWI, ADC maps

Differential Diagnosis

Space-Occupying CNS Mass in HIV+ Patient (seen in 10-12% of cases)
- Toxoplasmosis (hyperintense on DWI)
- Lymphoma (positive 201Tl-SPECT; most solitary mass lesions are lymphoma, especially if subependymal)
- Fungal infection, TB, syphilis
- Astrocytoma (rare)
- Kaposi sarcoma (skull, scalp involvement)

HIV

Pathology

<u>General</u>
- Etiology-Pathogenesis
  - Invasion of CNS by HIV-1 occurs at time of primary infection
  - Inflammatory (T-cell) reaction with vasculitis, leptomeningitis
  - Immune activation of parenchyma (increased microglial cells, upregulation of some antigens, production of cytokines)
- Epidemiology
  - 30% of AIDS patients have neurologic complications
  - HIV encephalitis occurs before opportunistic infections, neoplasms; prevalence unrelated to disease stage
  - Opportunistic infections or lymphoma only in brain in 31% of persons with fully developed AIDS, brain + other in 13%
  - Multiple CNS opportunistic infections + lymphoma in 4%
  - Cerebrovascular disease in 23% (seen at all stages), frank infarction in 18%

<u>Gross Pathologic or Surgical Features</u>
- Early: White matter pallor
- Late: Neocortical infection, atrophy

<u>Microscopic Features</u>
- HIVE
  - Perivascular accumulations of microglia, macrophages
  - Giant cells
- HIV leukoencephalopathy
  - Diffuse myelin loss
  - Astroglial proliferation
  - Macrophage infiltration

Clinical Issues

<u>Presentation</u>
- Variable (e.g., retinitis; myelitis/polyradiculopathy; encephalitis with HIV-associated dementia complex)

<u>Treatment & Prognosis</u>
- Biopsy focal mass if atypical neuroimaging features

Selected References
1. Thurnher MM et al: Primary central nervous system lymphoma in AIDS: a wider spectrum of CT and MRI findings. Neuroradiol 43: 29-35, 2001
2. Yin EZ et al: Primary immunodeficiency disorders in pediatric patients: Clinical features and imaging findings. AJR 176: 1541-52, 2001
3. Graham CB et al: Screening CT of the brain determined by CD4 count in HIV-positive patients presenting with headache. AJNR 21: 451-4, 2000

Tuberculosis (TB)

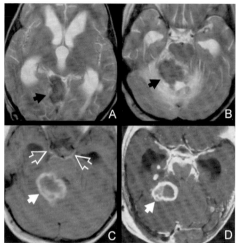

MR scans show TB granuloma with profoundly hypointense center on T2WI (A, B, black arrows), peripheral enhancement (C, D, white arrows). TB meningitis causes extensive cisternal enhancement, obstructive hydrocephalus. Both CNIIIs enhance (C, open arrows) (Courtesy K. Magnus).

Key Facts
- High prevalence, resurgence due to AIDS, drug-resistant strains
- In some countries TB represents 10%-30% of intracranial masses
- CNS TB often mimics other benign, malignant diseases
- Meningitis is most common manifestation

Imaging Findings
<u>General Features</u>
- Two different but related processes
  - Tuberculous meningitis (TBM)
  - Tuberculoma
- Best diagnostic sign= Basilar meningitis + extracerebral TB (e.g., pulmonary)

<u>CT Findings</u>
- TBM
  - May be normal early (10%-15%)
  - Isodense exudate effaces CSF spaces
  - Fills basal cisterns/sulci, enhances intensely
- Tuberculoma
  - Solitary or multiple
  - Hypo-, hyperdense round/lobulated mass +/- edema
  - Solid or ring-enhancing
  - Ca++ uncommon; "target sign" (central Ca++ surrounded by enhancing rim **not** pathognomonic for TB)

<u>MR Findings</u>
- TBM
  - Basal exudate isointense on T1-, hyperintense on T2WI
  - Enhances strongly, may have nodular components
  - Punctate/linear basal ganglia enhancement = vasculitis

49

Tuberculosis (TB)

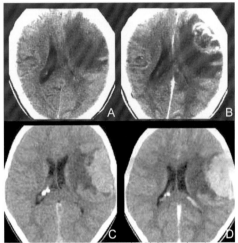

Two cases of TB mimicking brain tumors. (A, B) Ring-enhancing mass resembles GBM. (C, D) Dural-based mass resembles meningioma (cases courtesy R. Ramakantan).

- Tuberculoma
  - Noncaseating granuloma
    - Hypo- on T1-, hyperintense on T2WI
    - Enhances homogeneously
  - Caseating granuloma
    - Rim slightly hyperintense on T1WI, hypointense on T2WI
    - Ring enhancement (single, multiple or conglomerate)

Associated Findings
- Hydrocephalus (70%), infarcts (up to 40%)
- TB spondylitis (Pott's disease)
  - Spine most frequent osseous site
  - Infection starts in vertebral body, spreads to other levels, disks, soft tissues (paraspinal "cold" abscess)
  - Bone collapse + relative disk sparing = gibbous deformity
- Other sites = otomastoiditis, calvarium (+/- dura)
- TB cervical adenitis
  - Child/young adult with pulmonary disease
  - Conglomerate nodal mass (central lucency, thick enhancing rim)
  - Ca++ nodes highly suggestive of TB

Other Imaging Modality Findings
- MRS: TB abscess has lipid, lactate but not amino acid resonances

Differential Diagnosis

TBM
- Meningitis (other infectious agents, tumor, etc.)
- Noninfectious inflammatory meningiopathy (sarcoid, etc.)

Tuberculoma
- Abscess, other granuloma or parasite
- Primary or metastatic neoplasm

Tuberculosis (TB)

Pathology
General
- Etiology-Pathogenesis
  - Almost always secondary to pulmonary TB
  - Bacteria disseminate in CSF
  - Hyperemia, inflammation extend to basal meninges
  - May involve perivascular spaces, cause vasculitis
- Epidemiology
  - Worldwide: 8-10 million cases annually, 3 million deaths
  - Reemerging disease (immigration from endemic areas, immunocompromised patients, etc.)
  - Rise in multi drug-resistant strains (MDR-TB)

Gross Pathologic or Surgical Features
- TBM: Thick cisternal exudate (also sulci, interhemispheric fissure)
- Tuberculoma
  - Can be noncaseating, caseating with solid center, or caseating with necrotic center
  - Lobulated mass with central caseating necrosis, thick rim

Microscopic Features
- TBM: Inflammatory cells, fragile neocapillaries
- Tuberculoma
  - Mature tuberculoma = central liquefied caseating material
  - Early capsule = peripheral zone of fibroblasts, epithelioid cells, Langerhans' giant cells, lymphocytes
  - Late capsule = thick collagen layer
  - Hyperintense rim = collagenous fibers; hypointense = inflammatory cellular infiltrates (epithelioid cells, lymphocytes)

Clinical Issues
Presentation
- Varies from mild meningitis with no neurologic deficit to comatose
- CSF positive on initial LP in <40%
- Mycobacteria grow slowly so culture takes 4-8 weeks

Treatment & Prognosis
- Untreated TBM can be fatal in 4-8 weeks

Selected References
1. Pui MH et al: Magnetic resonance imaging findings in tuberculous meningoencephalitis. Can Assoc Radiol. J 52: 43-9, 2001
2. Harisinghani MG et al: Tuberculosis from head to toe. RadioGraphics 20: 449-70, 2000
3. Kim TK et al: Intracranial tuberculoma: Comparison of MR with pathologic findings. AJNR 16: 1903-8, 1995

Cysticercosis, Other Parasites

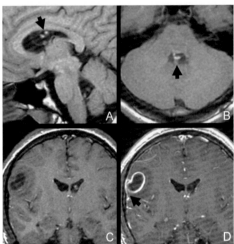

Cysticercosis with multiple intraventricular cysts (A, B, arrows). The "parenchymal" cyst (C, D) actually is extra-axial, lying within an enlarged sulcus. Note meningeal enhancement (D, arrow)(case courtesy N.Baldwin).

Key Facts
- Cysticercosis is most common, most widely disseminated parasitic infection in the world
- Brain infection (neurocysticercosis, NCC) found in 60%-90% of cases
- Most common cause of epilepsy in endemic areas
- Imaging findings vary with development stage
- **Complex conglomerated parasitic cysts of any etiology may mimic brain tumor!!**

Imaging Findings
General Features
- Best diagnostic sign = cyst with "dot" inside
- Imaging varies with development stage, host response
- Most common
  - Rounded or ovoid cyst, variable inflammation
  - Solitary in 20%-50%
  - When multiple, usually small number of cysts
  - Disseminated form ("miliary" NCC) rare
- Most common location = convexity subarachnoid spaces
- Inflammatory response around cyst may seal sulcus, make lesions appear intra-axial
- Other locations = parenchyma > ventricles > basal cisterns

CT Findings
- Vesicular stage (viable larva)
  - Smooth, thin-walled cyst rarely > 5-15 mm diameter
  - "Dot" within cyst = protoscolex
  - No (or mild) wall enhancement
  - No surrounding edema
- Colloidal vesicular stage (degenerating larva)
  - Hyperdense fluid
  - Thicker ring-enhancing fibrous capsule

Cysticercosis, Other Parasites

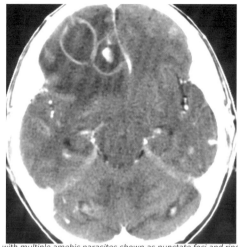

CECT scan with multiple amebic parasites shown as punctate foci and ring-enhancing cysts with nodules.

- ○ Surrounding edema
- Granular nodular (healing) stage
  - ○ Involuting enhancing nodule
  - ○ Edema mild, decreasing
- Nodular calcified (healed) stage
  - ○ Shrunken, calcified nodule

MR Findings (Degenerating Larvae)
- T1WI: Cyst hypo-, nodule isointense
- T2WI: Hyperintense cyst, edema
- FLAIR: Hyperintense, delineates scolex, useful for detecting intraventricular cysts
- Cyst wall, reactive fibrosis may enhance intensely

Other Parasitic Diseases
- Echinococcosis: Large uni- or multilocular cyst +/- detached germinal membrane, daughter cysts, no perilesional edema
- Schistosomiasis: Granulomatous encephalitis (hyperintense mass with enhancing dots along more linear area)
- Trichinosis: Eosinophilic meningoencephalitis, vascular thrombi and infarcts
- Paragonimiasis: In chronic stage, round and ovoid Ca++ in mass can resemble neoplasm
- Malaria: Punctate and ring hemorrhages, infarcts, cerebral edema (predilection for basal ganglia, cortex)
- Trypanosomiasis: Meningoencephalitis, organisms in VRSs cause brain edema, congestion, scattered petechial hemorrhages
- Sparganosis: Conglomerate, multicystic mass with surrounding edema may mimic neoplasm
- Amebic encephalitis: Meningoencephalitis; single or multiple focal, punctate, nodular or ring-enhancing masses

Cysticercosis, Other Parasites

Differential Diagnosis
NCC: Variable, Depending on Stage
- Other parasitic cysts
- TB

Parasitic Granulomas
- Neoplasm

Pathology
General
- General Path Comments
  - Findings depend on number, size, stage of infection
- Etiology-Pathogenesis-Pathophysiology
  - NCC caused by larval form of pig tapeworm, T.solium
  - Man is accidental intermediate host
    - Fecal-oral most common route of infection
    - Ingestion of eggs >> contaminated pork
- Epidemiology
  - NCC most common parasitic infection worldwide
  - Endemic in many countries
  - Increased travel, immigration have spread disease widely

Gross Pathologic, Surgical Features
- Usually small colorless cyst with invaginated scolex

Microscopic Features
- Cyst wall has 3 distinct layers
  - Outer (cuticular) layer
  - Middle cellular (pseudoepithelial) layer
  - Inner reticular (fibrillary) layer
- Scolex has rostellum with hooklets, muscular suckers
- Variable inflammatory reaction

Clinical Issues
Presentation
- Varies with organism, development stage, host immune response
- NCC asymptomatic until larvae degenerate
- NCC is most common cause of epilepsy in endemic areas

Natural History
- Variable
- Some parasitic infections (e.g., echinococcosis) develop slowly over many years

Selected References
1. Sabel M et al: Intracerebral neurocysticercosis mimicking glioblastoma multiforme. Neuroradiol 43: 227-30, 2001
2. Noujaim SE et al: CT and MR imaging of neurocysticercosis. AJR 173: 1485-90, 1999
3. Pittella JEH: Neurocysticercosis. Brain Pathol 7: 681-93, 1997

Post-Infection (ADEM)

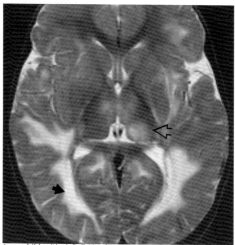

Axial T2WI in a child with A.D.E.M. shows lesions in both the gray matter nuclei (open arrow) and confluent hyperintensity in the periventricular white matter (black arrow).

Key Facts
- ADEM most common para/post-infectious disorder
- Triggered by inflammatory response to viral infections, vaccinations
- Children > adults but can affect all ages
- Solitary lesion may mimic neoplasm

Imaging Findings
General Features
- Severe acute demyelination
- Usually monophasic
- Imaging findings often lag behind clinical presentation, resolution
- Best diagnostic sign = multifocal WM/basal ganglia lesions 10 days-2 weeks following infection/vaccination

CT Findings
- NECT
  - Initial CT normal in 40%
  - Low-density, flocculent, asymmetric lesions
  - +/- Mild mass effect
- CECT
  - Multifocal punctate or ring-enhancing lesions
  - Solitary lesion can mimic neoplasm

MR Findings
- Initial imaging often normal but more sensitive than CT
  - Findings may be associated with recovery > decline
- T2WI, FLAIR
  - Multifocal punctate/large flocculent hyperintensities
  - Bilateral but asymmetric (involve peripheral WM/GM)
  - Do not usually involve callososeptal interface
- Contrast-enhanced T1WI
  - Punctate or ring-enhancing

Post-Infection (ADEM)

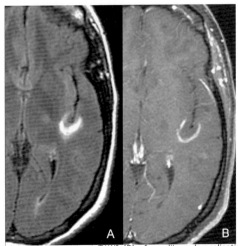

Axial FLAIR (A) and post-contrast T1WI (B) of a solitary demyelinating lesion in A.D.E.M. Note the incomplete ("horseshoe") pattern of enhancement.

- o Cranial nerve(s) may enhance
- Rare manifestations of ADEM
  - o Hemorrhagic, hyperacute variant
  - o Bilateral striatal necrosis (usually in infants, may be reversible)

Other Modality Findings
- DWI: Variable
- MRS: NAA transiently low, choline normal

Imaging Recommendations
- Acute and convalescent contrast-enhanced MR best
- Limited rapid interval follow-up may be provided by "FLAIR" alone

Differential Diagnosis
Multiple Sclerosis
- Predilection for periventricular WM (callososeptal interface)
- Lesions often more symmetric than ADEM
- Relapsing-remitting course common

Autoimmune-Mediated Vasculitis
- Multifocal GM/WM lesions
  - o Bilateral, usually cortical/subcortical, basal ganglia
  - o Ring-enhancing lesions mimics infection (e.g., toxoplasmosis)

High Grade Glioma
- "Tumefactive" demyelination may occur with both MS, ADEM
- MRS shows elevated choline, decreased NAA

Pathology
General
- Genetics
  - o No sex predominance ADEM
  - o In children, MS has no sex predominance but adolescent/young adults female:male = 2-3:1

Post-Infection (ADEM)

- ▪ May implicate hormonal role
- Etiology-Pathogenesis-Pathophysiology
  - ○ Autoimmune-mediated demyelination
  - ○ Specific infections, manifestations include
    - ▪ Mumps (deafness)
    - ▪ Streptococci (Sydenham's chorea)
    - ▪ Mycoplasma (bilateral hippocampal sclerosis)
    - ▪ Chickenpox (cerebellitis)
    - ▪ Ebstein-Barr (basal ganglia foci)
    - ▪ Influenza A (acute necrotizing encephalopathy, thalamic/basal ganglia)
- Epidemiology
  - ○ Unknown, increasingly reported

Gross Pathologic, Surgical Features
- Usually none

Microscopic Features
- Acute myelin breakdown
- Lymphocytic infiltrates
- Relative axonal preservation
- Atypical astrogliosis

Clinical Issues
Presentation
- Peak age 3-5 years (can occur at any age)
- Usually (but not always) preceded by prodromal phase
  - ○ Fever, malaise
  - ○ Myalgia
- Multifocal neurological symptoms
  - ○ Hemiparesis, cranial nerve palsies common
  - ○ Decreased consciousness (varies from lethargy to coma, convulsions)
  - ○ Behavioral changes
- CSF often abnormal (leukocytosis, elevated protein)

Natural History
- Variable
  - ○ Mortality 10%-30%
  - ○ 20%-30% neurologic sequelae
  - ○ 50%-60% complete recovery
  - ○ Relapses rare
    - ▪ "Relapsing disseminated encephalomyelitis"
    - ▪ May not be a separate entity from relapsing-remitting MS
- Typically delay between symptom onset, imaging findings

Treatment & Prognosis
- Immunomodulatory therapy

Selected References
1. Bizzi A et al, Quantitative proton MR spectroscopic imaging in acute disseminated encephalomyelitis. AJNR 22: 1125-30, 2001
2. Honkaniemi J et al: Delayed MR imaging changes in acute disseminated encephalomyelitis. AJNR 22: 1117-24, 2001
3. Dale RC et al: Acute disseminated encephalomyelitis, multiphasic disseminated encephalyomyelitis and multiple sclerosis in children. Brain 12:2407-22, 2000

ANEURYSMS

Aneurysmal Hemorrhage (aSAH)

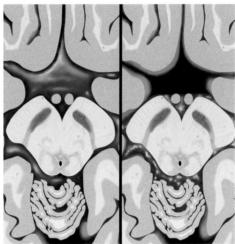

Axial graphics depict patterns of cisternal blood in aneurysmal SAH (aSAH, left) and perimesencephalic nonaneurysmal SAH (pnSAH, right).

Key Facts
- Most common cause of SAH is **trauma** (not aneurysm rupture)
- Most common complication of aSAH = vasospasm
- Perimesencephalic nonaneurysmal subarachnoid hemorrhage (pnSAH) = benign entity with CT features distinct from aSAH

Imaging Findings
General Features
- aSAH = blood in suprasellar/sylvian/interhemispheric cisterns
- pnSAH = "pretruncal" hemorrhage (in front of pons, around midbrain)

CT Findings
- aSAH = high attenuation in basal subarachnoid spaces
  - Acute aSAH 95% positive NECT scan in first 24h
  - Sensitivity for aSAH decreases with time, < 50% by 1 week
- pnSAH
  - High attenuation anterior to midbrain, in ambient cisterns
  - Minimal/no extension into sylvian, interhemispheric fissures
  - In > 90% of pnSAH, no SAH visible at 1 week

MR Findings
- Acute SAH = "dirty" CSF
  - Iso- with brain on T1WI, hyperintense on T2WI
  - High signal intensity on FLAIR (**not** pathognomonic for SAH)
  - Low signal intensity on T2* sequences
- Chronic SAH
  - "Superficial siderosis" (hypointense line along brain, spinal cord, cranial nerves on T2WI, T2*)

Other Modality Findings
- CTA/MRA/DSA
  - Negative in 15%-20% of aSAH
  - 5% prevalence of vertebrobasilar aneurysm in pnSAH

Aneurysmal Hemorrhage (aSAH)

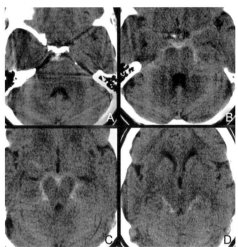

NECT scans show typical pnSAH with focal prepontine, interpeduncular, and perimesencephalic subarachnoid blood. DSA was normal.

- o Multiple aneurysms 20%-33% (largest/irregular aneurysm most likely to have ruptured)

Imaging Recommendations
- • NECT scan
  - o If positive, CTA (excellent for aneurysms > 3 mm)
    - ▪ If CTA positive, surgery; consider DSA (endovascular Rx)
    - ▪ If pnSAH pattern + negative CTA, DSA could be omitted
  - o If negative, fluoroscopy-guided lumbar puncture
    - ▪ 12h post-SAH for xanthochromia approach 100% sensitivity
    - ▪ 1000 cells/mm^3 includes almost all true aSAH cases, limits false-positive rate to < 5%

Differential Diagnosis
aSAH vs. pnSAH
- • Pattern, distribution of SAH

Other Causes of SAH
- • Occult trauma, dissection
- • Vascular malformation (cavernous malformation, spinal dAVF)
- • Vascular neoplasm (e.g., ependymoma)

Sulcal High Signal on FLAIR
- • Infectious/inflammatory meningitis
- • Carcinomatous meningitis
- • Propofol anesthetic, supplemental oxygen
- • Artifact (multifactorial; spurious high CSF signal)
- • Gadolinium in CSF (renal failure)

Pathology
General
- • Etiology-Pathogenesis
  - o pnSAH: Ruptured perimesencephalic/prepontine vein

Aneurysmal Hemorrhage (aSAH)

- Epidemiology
  - aSAH causes 2%-4% of "strokes"
  - pnSAH accounts for 20%-70% of angiogram-negative aSAH

Gross Pathologic or Surgical Features
- Clotted blood in basal cisterns

Microscopic Features
- Early: Arterial smooth muscle contraction, vasoconstriction
- Late: Smooth muscle necrosis, endothelial desquamation, apoptosis

Staging or Grading Criteria
- Clinical: Hunt and Hess
  - 0 = unruptured
  - 1 = asymptomatic or minimal headache, nuchal rigidity
  - 2 = moderate HA, no deficit other than CN palsy
  - 3 = drowsy, mild focal deficit
  - 4 = stuporous, hemiparesis, early decerebrate
  - 5 = deep coma, moribund
- CT: Fisher score
  - 0 = unruptured
  - 1 = no blood
  - 2 = diffuse < 1mm thick
  - 3 = local lot or > 2mm
  - 4 = ICH or IVH

Clinical Issues

Presentation
- Similar for aSAH, pnSAH (headache, meningismus, etc.)

Natural History of aSAH
- 50% mortality
- 13.6% rebleed within first 24h
- Vasospasm = major cause of delayed morbidity, mortality
  - 70%-90% prevalence during first 2 weeks following SAH
    - Caused by prostacyclin release, decreased iNO
    - Onset 3-5 days after aSAH, maximal at 5-8 days
    - Gradual resolution
  - 50% develop ischemic neurologic deficits
- Chronic hydrocephalus develops in 10%-25% of cases

Natural History of pnSAH
- Benign clinical course, no rebleeding

Treatment & Prognosis
- aSAH: Locate, clip/coil ruptured aneurysm
- pnSAH: No further studies are usually required

Selected References
1. Eskey CJ et al: Fluoroscopy-guided lumbar puncture: Decreased frequency of traumatic tap and implications for the assessment of CT-negative acute subarachnoid hemorrhage. AJNR 22: 571-6, 2001
2. Ohkuma H et al: Incidence and significance of early aneurysmal rebleeding. Stroke 32: 1176-80, 2001
3. Ruigrok YM et al: Perimesencephalic hemorrhagic and CT angiography. Stroke 31: 2976-83, 2000

Saccular Aneurysm

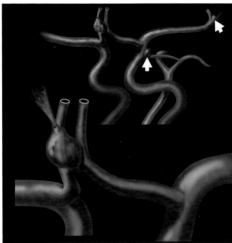

Graphic depiction of the circle of Willis shows a large, lobulated, aCoA aneurysm with rupture into the subarachnoid space. Unruptured aneurysms are also depicted at the MCA and PCoA (white arrows).

Key Facts
- Aneurysm formation multifactorial
- Genetics play increasingly recognized role
- Subarachnoid hemorrhage (aSAH) most common presentation
- Size most important (but not only) factor in rupture risk

Imaging Findings
General Features
- Best diagnostic sign= round, lobulated or bleblike outpouching
- Usually arises from vessel bifurcation > lateral wall
- Involves short segment of vessel wall

CT Findings
- Ruptured = high density blood in basal cisterns (see "aSAH")
- Patent aneurysm
  - Well-delineated round/lobulated extra-axial mass
  - Slightly hyperdense to brain (may have mural Ca++)
  - Enhances strongly
- Partially/completely thrombosed aneurysm
  - Moderately hyperdense (Ca++ common)
  - Patent lumen enhances

MR Findings
- +/- Subarachnoid blood (see "aSAH")
- Patent aneurysm (signal varies)
  - 50% have "flow void" (high velocity signal loss)
  - Iso/heterogeneous signal, incomplete delineation
    - Slow/turbulent flow
    - Saturation effects, phase dispersion
- Partially/completely thrombosed aneurysm
  - Signal depends on age(s) of clot
  - Often hyperintense on T1-, hypointense on T2WI

Saccular Aneurysm

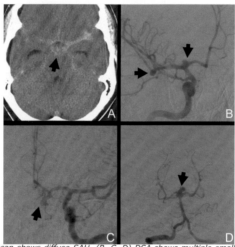

(A) CECT scan shows diffuse SAH. (B, C, D) DSA shows multiple small aneurysms (arrows). The large, irregular, ACoA aneurysm (C, arrow) is the one that ruptured.

- o   May be laminated with very hypointense rim
- o   Patent lumen enhances

Other Modality Findings
- • Role of DSA/CTA/MRA
  - o   Delineate aneurysm, define neck, detect multiple aneurysms
  - o   Identify perforating arteries that may arise from dome
  - o   Assess potential for collateral circulation
- • Findings
  - o   Round/lobulated, focal outpouching, may have apical "tit"
  - o   Narrow or broad-based

Imaging Recommendations
- • CTA, MRA excellent screening tools for aneurysms > 3-4 mm

Differential Diagnosis

Small Patent Aneurysm
- • Vessel loop (use multiple projections)
- • Infundibulum (< 3 mm, conical, small PCoA from apex)

Thrombosed Aneurysm
- • Hemorrhagic neoplasm, thrombosed vascular malformation

Pathology

General
- • Genetics (increasingly recognized role)
  - o   Abnormal expression/functional polymorphism of some genes
    - ▪ Endoglin, MMP-9
    - ▪ Overexpression of other genes encoding extracellular matrix components (e.g., collagen, elastin)
  - o   Hereditary, connective tissue disorders
    - ▪ Ehlers-Danlos type IV, NF-1
    - ▪ Fibromuscular dysplasia
    - ▪ Autosomal dominant polycystic kidney disease (10%)

Saccular Aneurysm

- o Familial intracranial aneurysms (no known heritable disorder)
    - • Occur in "clusters" (two first-order relatives)
    - • 10% prevalence (vs. 1%-2% autopsy prevalence)
    - • Significantly younger patients
    - • Up to 20% of all aSAH
- • Etiology-Pathogenesis-Pathophysiology
    - o Flow-related "bioengineering fatigue" in vessel wall
    - o Abnormal vascular hemodynamics
        - • Arises at areas of high biomechanical stress
        - • Abnormal slipstream vectors
        - • Higher/disturbed flow, increased pulsatility
- • Epidemiology
    - o From 1.22/100,000 person-yr (age 0-34) to 44.47/100,000 person-yr (age 65-74)
        - • Women > men (especially with multiple aneurysms)
    - o Rare in children
        - • 1%-2% of all aneurysms
        - • Different location (ICA bifurcation, M2 MCA)
    - o 20% multiple

Gross Pathologic or Surgical Features
- • Round/lobulated sac, thin or thick wall, +/- SAH

Microscopic Features
- • Disrupted/absent internal elastic lamina
- • Muscle layer absent
- • May have "tit" of fragile adventitia

Clinical Issues
Presentation
- • Intracranial hemorrhage 60%-85%
    - o Headache (often "thunderclap")
- • Other: "Migraine," cranial neuropathy, TIA, seizure

Natural History (rupture risk)
- • Size (small if < 10mm, high if > 25 mm)
- • Shape (multilobed, "tit", aspect ratio > 1.6)
- • "Perianeurysmal environment" (contact with other structures)?
- • Other (hypertension, female gender, smoking)

Selected References
1. Proust F et al: Pediatric cerebral aneurysms. J Neurosurg 94: 733-9, 2001
2. White PM et al: Intracranial aneurysms: CTA and MRA for detection. Radiol 219: 739-49, 2001
3. Menghini VV et al: Clinical manifestations and survival rates among patients with saccular intracranial aneurysms. Neurosurg 49: 251-8, 2001

Fusiform Aneurysm (FA)

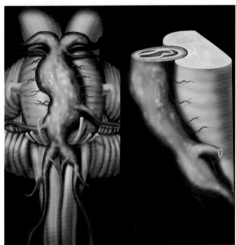

Graphic depicts atherosclerotic fusiform aneurysm of the vertebrobasilar system.

Key Facts
- FA less common than saccular aneurysm
- FAs involve long, nonbranching vessel segments
- Can be acute (dissecting aneurysm) or chronic (ASVD, nonatherosclerotic vasculopathy)

Imaging Findings
General Features
- Best diagnostic sign= long segment fusiform or ovoid arterial dilatation
CT Findings
- NECT: Hyperdense; Ca++ common
- CECT: Lumen enhances strongly, intramural clot doesn't
MR Findings
- Ectatic vessel +/- more focal aneurysmal outpouching
- Mixed signal intensity common, varies with
  - Flow velocity, direction, turbulence
    - Slow flow seen as high signal deep into imaged sections
  - Presence, age of mural hematoma
    - Often hyperintense on T1WI, hypointense rim on T2WI
    - Clot may be laminated (layers of organized thrombus at different stages of evolution)
- Residual lumen enhances strongly
Other Modality Findings
- MRA
  - Precontrast 3D-TOF may be inadequate because of
    - Flow saturation effects
    - Intravoxel phase dispersion
  - Giant FA usually requires dynamic contrast-enhanced sequences for accurate delineation
- DSA/CTA
  - Exaggerated arterial ectasia(s)

Fusiform Aneurysm (FA)

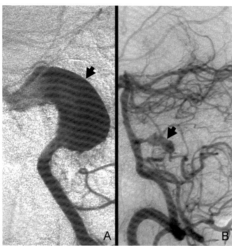

(A) Lateral vertebrobasilar angiogram shows an atherosclerotic fusiform aneurysm (arrow). (B) Lateral vertebrobasilar angiogram in a 21-year-old male with collagen-vascular disease shows a nonatherosclerotic fusiform AICA aneurysm (arrow).

- o   More focal fusiform or even saccular enlargement may occur
- o   Can be solitary or multifocal

Differential Diagnosis
Vertebrobasilar Dolichoectasia
- •   Older patient
- •   Changes of ASVD in other vessels
- •   Ectasia often extends into branches
Giant Serpentine Aneurysm
- •   Large, partially thrombosed mass
- •   Distal branches arise from aneurysm dome
- •   Lacks definable neck
- •   May be indistinguishable from FA
Nonatherosclerotic Fusiform Vasculopathy
- •   Younger patient
- •   History of inherited vasculopathy, immune disorder

Pathology
General
- •   FAs can be atherosclerotic, nonatherosclerotic
- •   Nonatherosclerotic fusiform and dissecting aneurysms
    - o   Type 1 = typical dissecting aneurysm
    - o   Type 2 = segmental ectasias
    - o   Type 3 = dolichoectatic dissecting aneurysms
    - o   Type 4 = atypically located saccular aneurysm (i.e., lateral wall, unrelated to branching zones)
- •   Genetics
    - o   Marfan syndrome: Mutation of fibrillin genes (FBN1)
- •   Etiology-Pathogenesis

Fusiform Aneurysm (FA)

- o Atherosclerosis usual cause of basilar FA in older adults
  - Lipid deposition is initial step
  - IEL, muscle layers become disrupted
  - Enhanced susceptibility to hemodynamic stress
- o Nonatherosclerotic fusiform aneurysms
  - IEL fragmentation is initial step
  - Immune deficiency (e.g., HIV)
  - Viral, other infectious agents (e.g., varicella)
  - Collagen vascular disorders (i.e., SLE)

Gross Pathologic or Surgical Features
- Focally dilated fusiform arterial ectasia(s)
- +/- ASVD

Microscopic Features
- Type 1 = widespread disruption of the IEL, no intimal thickening
- Type 2 = extended and/or fragmented IEL with intimal thickening
- Type 3 = IEL fragmentation, multiple dissections of thickened intima, organized thrombus
- Type 4 = absent IEL, muscular layer

Clinical Issues
Presentation
- Pain, SAH
- TIAs, cranial neuropathy

Natural History
- Type 1: Rebleed common
- Type 2: Benign clinical course
- Type 3: Slow but progressive enlargement
- Type 4: Rerupture risk high

Treatment & Prognosis
- Often combined surgical, endovascular
- 80% of giant "unclippable" aneurysms dead/disabled at 5 years

Selected References
1. Jager HR et al: Contrast-enhanced MR angiography of intracranial giant aneurysms. AJNR 21: 1900-7, 2000
2. Nakatomi H et al: Clinicopathological study of intracranial fusiform and dolichoectatic aneurysms. Stroke 31: 896-900, 2000
3. Mizutani T et al: Proposed classification of nonatherosclerotic cerebral fusiform and dissecting aneurysms. Neurosurg 45: 253-60, 1999

"Blood Blisterlike" Aneurysm

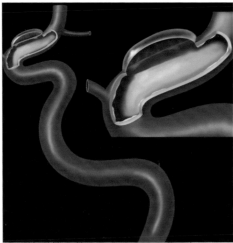

Graphic depicts a blood blisterlike aneurysm arising along the greater curvature of the supraclinoid ICA. The aneurysm wall consists of a thin, fibrous cap.

Key Facts
- Rare but important source of aneurysmal SAH (aSAH)
- Focal arterial wall defect covered only with fibrous tissue
- Tends to rupture earlier, at smaller size than saccular aneurysm

Imaging Findings
General Features
- Best diagnostic sign= small, broad-based, hemispherical bulge
CT Findings
- aSAH
MR Findings
- aSAH, otherwise usually negative
- +/- Seen on high-resolution MRA
Other Modality Findings
- DSA
    - Initial angiogram often read as normal ("angiographically negative SAH")
    - Slight irregularity/small focal bulge of arterial wall may be only finding!

Differential Diagnosis
Saccular Aneurysm
- Usually arises at arterial bifurcation/ branching point
- Round, lobulated
PCoA Infundibulum
- Funnel-shaped
- PCoA arises from apex

Pathology
General
- Blister-like pseudoaneurysm

"Blood Blisterlike" Aneurysm

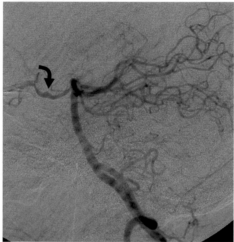

Lateral vertebrobasilar angiogram in a patient with typical aneurysmal SAH shows a small, broad-based outpouching along the PCoA (curved arrow). Ruptured blisterlike aneurysm was found at surgery.

- Etiology-Pathogenesis-Pathophysiology
  - ○ Unknown
  - ○ Atherosclerosis with ulceration, hematoma formation?

Gross Pathologic or Surgical Features
- Broad-based bulge
- Arises from unbranched (lateral) arterial wall
- Can occur anywhere
  - ○ Greater curvature of supraclinoid ICA is most common site
  - ○ Posterior circulation not uncommon location

Microscopic Features
- Dome composed of fibrous tissue/adventitia
- No other vessel wall elements
- Significant arteriosclerosis in parent vessel common

Clinical Issues
Presentation
- aSAH

Natural History
- Tend to rupture earlier, at smaller size than saccular aneurysm

Treatment & Prognosis
- High surgical mortality/morbidity
  - ○ Small size, very thin wall, wide base
  - ○ Avulse readily, intraoperative rupture common
  - ○ Parent vessel lumen easily compromised
  - ○ Wrapping may permit regrowth
- Options: "Trapping" or stenting

Selected References
1. Kobayashi S et al: Blisterlike aneurysms. J Neurosurg 91: 164-6, 1999
2. Charbel FT et al: Distal internal carotid artery pseudoaneurysms. Neurosurg 45: 643-9, 1999
3. Abe M et al: Blood blisterlike aneurysms of the internal carotid artery. J Neurosurg 89: 419-24, 1998

VASCULAR MALFORMATIONS

AV Malformation (AVM)

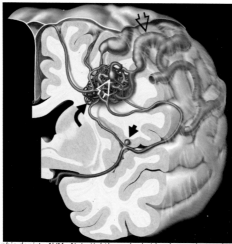

Coronal graphic depicts AVM. Note tightly packed nidus (curved arrow) with intranidal aneurysm (open white arrow), "pedicle" aneurysm (black arrow), and venous varices (open black arrow).

Key Facts
- Most common symptomatic cerebral vascular malformation (CVM)
- AVMs have dysregulated angiogenesis, undergo continued vascular remodeling

Imaging Findings
General Features
- Tightly packed mass of enlarged vascular channels
- No normal brain inside
- Best diagnostic sign= "bag of black worms" (flow voids) with minimal/no mass effect on MR

CT Findings
- NECT (may be normal with very small AVM)
  - Iso/hyperdense serpentine vessels
  - Ca++ in 25%-30%
  - Variable hemorrhage
- CECT: Strong enhancement

MR Findings
- Varies with flow rate, direction, presence/age of hemorrhage
- "Honeycomb" of "flow voids"
- Nidus contains little or no brain

Other Modality Findings
- DSA
  - Delineates internal angioarchitecture (superselective best)
  - Findings
    - Little or no mass effect
    - Enlarged arteries
    - Nidus of tightly packed vessels
    - AV shunt ("early draining vein")

AV Malformation (AVM)

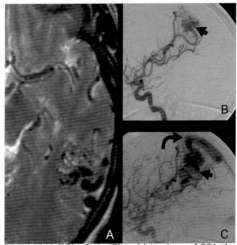

(A) T2WI shows typical AVM. Early (B) and late phase of DSA show the nidus (arrows) and early draining vein (curved arrow).

- CTA/MRA
  - Helpful for gross depiction of flow, post-embo/XRT
  - 3D contrast-enhanced studies improve delineation

Differential Diagnosis

Patent AVM vs. Glioblastoma With AV Shunting
- GBM enhances, has mass effect
- Some parenchyma between vessels

Thrombosed ("Cryptic") AVM Versus
- Cavernous angioma
- Calcified neoplasm
- Oligodendroglioma
- Low-grade astrocytoma

Pathology

General
- General Path Comments
  - 85% supratentorial; 15% posterior fossa
  - Sporadic AVMs are solitary
- Genetics
  - No specific mutations for sporadic AVMs
  - Multiple AVMs (2% of cases)
    - HHT 1 (chromosome 9, 12 mutations)
    - Cerebral AV metameric syndromes (Wyburn-Mason) have orbit/maxillofacial, intracranial AVMs
- Etiology-Pathogenesis
  - Old: Retention of primitive embryonic vascular network?
  - New: Dysregulated angiogenesis
    - VEGFs, receptors mediate endothelial proliferation, migration
    - Cytokine receptors mediate vascular maturation, remodeling

AV Malformation (AVM)

- Epidemiology
  - Prevalence of sporadic AVMs = .04-.52%

Gross Pathologic or Surgical Features
- Central nidus plus arterial feeders, venous outflow

Microscopic Features (Wide Phenotypic Spectrum)
- Feeding arteries, draining veins
  - Mature vessels (may have some wall thickening)
- Nidus
  - Thin-walled dysplastic vessels (no capillary bed)
    - Lack intact tight junctions, subendothelial support
    - Loss of normal contractile properties
  - Conglomeration of numerous AV shunts
  - No normal brain (may have some gliosis)
- Associated abnormalities
  - Flow-related aneurysm on feeding artery 10%-15%
  - Intranidal "aneurysm" > 50%
  - Hemorrhage, +/- Ca++

Staging or Grading Criteria (Spetzler-Martin)
- Size
  - Small (<3 cm)   1
  - Medium (3-6 cm)   2
  - Large (>6 cm)   3
- Location
  - Noneloquent   0
  - Eloquent   1
- Venous drainage
  - Superficial only   0
  - Deep   1

Clinical Issues

Presentation
- Peak presentation = 20-40y (25% by age 15)
  - Hemorrhage 50%
  - Seizures 25%
  - Neurologic deficit 20%-25%

Natural History
- Hemorrhage 2%-4%/year, cumulative
- Spontaneous obliteration rare (1%-3% of cases)

Treatment & Prognosis
- Embolization, radiosurgery, surgery

Selected References
1. Warren DJ et al: Cerebral arteriovenous malformations: Comparison of novel MRA techniques and conventional catheter angiography. Neurosurg 48: 973-83, 2001
2. Uranishi R et al: Vascular smooth muscle cell differentiation in human cerebral vascular malformations. Neurosurg 49: 671-80, 2001
3. Berman MF et al: The epidemiology of brain arteriovenous malformations. Neurosurg 47: 389-97, 2000

Dural AV Shunts (dAVSs)

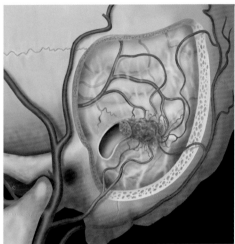

Graphic with cutaway of transverse sinus depicts a dAVS. The sinus is thrombosed and numerous "crack-like" vessels are present in the sinus wall. Supply is from dural branches of both ECA and ICA.

Key Facts
- dAVSs also known as dural arteriovenous fistulae (dAVFs)
- Cluster of numerous "micro" AV shunts inside dural sinus wall
- Most are acquired, express active angiogenesis
- Clinical manifestations vary with location, presence of venous hypertension

Imaging Findings
General Features
- Adult-type dAVS
  - Best diagnostic sign = network of tiny "crack-like" vessels in thrombosed dural sinus
- Infantile dAVS (rare)
  - Best diagnostic sign = multiple high-flow shunts involving different dural sinuses

CT Findings
- NECT: Often normal
- CECT
  - May be normal with small shunts
  - +/- Serpentine feeders, enlarged dural sinus
  - Enlarged superior ophthalmic vein (with CCF)

MR Findings
- May be normal
- Thrombosed transverse/sigmoid (TS/SS) sinus contains numerous flow voids from "micro" fistulae ("crack-like" vessels)

Other Modality Findings
- DSA
  - Most common = TS or SS dAVS
    - Dural sinus often thrombosed
    - Flow reversal in dural sinus/cortical correlates with progressive symptoms, risk of hemorrhage

Dural AV Shunts (dAVSs)

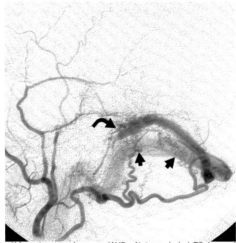

External carotid angiogram shows a dAVF. Note occluded TS (curved arrow) and numerous enlarged dural, transosseous feeders (black arrows) supplying the lesion in the sinus wall.

- Tortuous engorged pial veins ("pseudophlebitic pattern") with venous congestion/hypertension (clinically aggressive)
  o Second most common = carotid-cavernous fistula (CCF)
    - Type A: Direct ICA-cavernous sinus shunt (not true dAVS)
    - Type B: Dural ICA branches-cavernous shunt
    - Type C: Dural ECA-cavernous shunt
    - Type D: ECA/ICA dural branches shunt to cavernous sinus
- MRA
  o May be negative with small or slow flow shunts
  o Gross depiction but doesn't delineate detailed angioarchitecture
- PET/SPECT: May show increased rCBV, decreased rCBF (venous ischemia)

Imaging Recommendations
- Screening MR with contrast
- DSA to delineate vascular supply, venous drainage

Differential Diagnosis
Mixed Pial-Dural AVM
- True pial supply to dAVS is rare
- Usually occurs with large posterior fossa dAVS
Vascular Neoplasm
- Acutely thrombosed dAVS may enhance, have edema/mass effect

Pathology
General
- General path comments
  o No true nidus
- Etiology-Pathogenesis-Pathophysiology
  o Most dAVSs are acquired
    - May be idiopathic

- Can occur in response to trauma, venous occlusion, or venous hypertension
  o Pathological activation of neoangiogenesis
    - Proliferating capillaries within granulation tissue in dural sinus obliterated by organized thrombi
    - Budding/proliferation of microvascular network in inner dura connects to plexus of thin-walled venous channels
    - High bFGF, VEGF expression in dAVSs
- Epidemiology
  o 10%-15% of all cerebrovascular malformations with AV shunting
  o Location: Can occur anywhere but usually near skull base

Gross Pathologic, Surgical Features
- Multiple enlarged dural feeders converge on dural sinus
- Collection of "crack-like" vessels in wall of thrombosed sinus

Clinical Issues
Presentation
- Varies with age, location, severity of AV shunting
- Common
  o Bruit, pulsatile tinnitus
  o Exophthalmos
  o Cranial neuropathy
- Uncommon
  o Progressive dementia
  o Parkinsonism
- Rare
  o Life-threatening congestive heart failure
  o Usually neonates, infants

Natural History
- Variable; can be aggressive with devastating hemorrhage
- Spontaneous closure rare

Treatment & Prognosis
- Endovascular
- Surgical resection
- Stereotaxic radiosurgery

Selected References
1. Kawaguchi T et al: Classification of venous ischaemia with MRI. J Clin Neurosci 8 (suppl 1): 82-8, 2001
2. Friedman JA et al: Results of combined stereotactic radiosurgery and transarterial embolization for dural arteriovenous fistulas of the transverse and sigmoid sinuses. J Neurosurg 94: 886-91, 2001
3. Uranishi R et al: Expression of angiogenic growth factors in dural arteriovenous fistula. J Neurosurg 91: 781-6, 1999

Venous "Angioma" (VA)

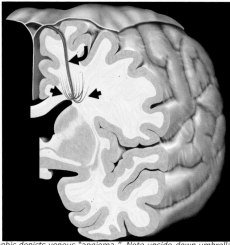

Coronal graphic depicts venous "angioma." Note upside-down umbrella appearance of prominent medullary veins ("Medusa head," black arrows) and single transcortical collector vein (curved arrow) draining into SSS.

Key Facts
- VAs consist of angiogenically mature elements, represent anatomic variants of normal venous drainage
- Most VAs are asymptomatic
- VAs may be histologically mixed (cavernous malformation)

Imaging Findings
General Features
- Umbrella-like collection of enlarged medullary (white matter) veins
- Near ventricle (frontal horn, fourth ventricle most common sites)
- Large "collector" vein drains into dural sinus or deep ependymal vein
- Best diagnostic sign = "Medusa head" (dilated white matter veins)

CT Findings
- NECT: Usually normal
- CECT: Numerous linear or dot-like enhancing foci
  - Converge on single enlarged tubular draining vein
    - Occasionally seen as linear structure in a single slice
    - More often appears as well-circumscribed round/ovoid enhancing areas on sequential sections

MR Findings
- Variable signal depending on size, flow
  - "Flow void" on T1-, T2WI
- Strong enhancement
- Stellate, tubular vessels converge on collector vein
- Collector vein drains into dural sinus/ependymal vein
- +/- Hemorrhage (from co-existing cavernous malformation)

Other Modality Findings
- DSA
  - Arterial phase normal
  - Capillary phase
    - Usually normal

Venous "Angioma" (VA)

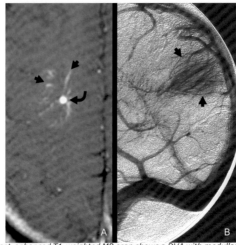

Axial contrast-enhanced T1-weighted MR scan shows a DVA with medullary tributaries (arrows) and collector vein (curved arrow). (B) Venous phase DSA shows typical "Medusa head" (arrows).

- Rarely VAs may have prominent vascular blush, A-V shunt
  - Venous phase: "Medusa head"

Differential Diagnosis
Vascular Neoplasm (e.g., GBM)
- Enlarged medullary veins
- Mass effect, usually enhances
Dural Sinus Occlusion With Venous Stasis
- Sinus thrombosis
- Medullary veins enlarge as collateral drainage
Demyelinating Disease (Rare)
- Active demyelination with prominent medullary veins

Pathology
General
- General Path Comments
  - Most common cerebral vascular malformation at autopsy
- Genetics
  - Mutations in chromosomes 1, 9
    - Encode for surface cell receptors
    - Tie-2 mutation results in missense activation, familial multiorgan venous malformations
  - Some inherited as autosomal dominant
- Embryology
  - Persistence of large embryonic white matter veins
- Etiology, pathogenesis
  - Do not express growth factors
  - Express structural proteins of mature angiogenesis
  - May represent extreme anatomic variant of otherwise normal venous drainage

Venous "Angioma" (VA)

- Epidemiology
  - 60% of cerebral vascular malformations
  - 2.5%-9% prevalence on contrast-enhanced MR scans
  - Usually solitary
- Associated abnormalities
  - Blue rubber bleb nevus syndrome
  - Sinus pericranii
  - Other cutaneous head and neck venous malformations
  - Sulcation-gyration disorders

Gross Pathologic or Surgical Features
- Radially oriented dilated medullary veins
- Separated by normal brain
- Enlarged transcortical or subependymal draining vein

Microscopic Features
- Enlarged but otherwise normal veins
- Normal brain without gliosis
- 20% have mixed histology, may hemorrhage

Clinical Issues

Presentation
- Usually asymptomatic, discovered incidentally at imaging
- Uncommon
  - Headache
  - Seizure (if associated with cortical dysplasia)
  - Hemorrhage with focal neurologic deficit (if associated with cavernous malformation)

Natural History
- Hemorrhage risk 0.15% per lesion-year, increased if
  - Stenosis or thrombosis of draining vein
  - Co-existing cavernous malformation

Treatment & Prognosis
- Solitary VA: None (attempt at removal may cause venous infarction)
- Histologically mixed VA: Determined by co-existing lesion

Selected References
1. Kilic T et al: Expression of structural proteins and angiogenic factors in cerebrovascular anomalies. Neurosurg 46: 1179-92, 2000
2. Komiyama M et al: Venous angiomas with arteriovenous shunts. Neurosurg 44: 1328-35, 1999
3. Naff NJ et al: A longitudinal study of patients with venous malformations. Neurol 50: 1709-14, 1998

Capillary Telangiectasia (CT)

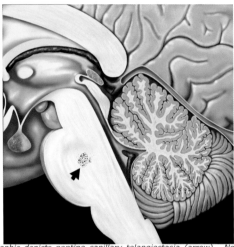

Sagittal graphic depicts pontine capillary telangiectasia (arrow). Note enlarged capillaries with normal brain between the dilated vessels.

Key Facts
- Most CTs are discovered incidentally at imaging or autopsy
- Clinically benign (unless histologically mixed with other malformation such as cavernous or venous malformation)
- CTs contain normal brain

Imaging Findings
General Features
- Small, poorly-demarcated lesion(s)
- Consists of dilated capillaries
- Contains normal brain
- No gross hemorrhage
- Midbrain, pons, medulla, spinal cord most common sites
- Best diagnostic sign = ill-defined lesion with faint "brush-like" enhancement

CT Findings
- Usually normal

MR Findings
- Solitary lesion
  - T1WI usually normal
  - 50% are hyperintense on T2WI, FLAIR
  - May be hypointense on T2* scan (slow intralesional blood flow permits desaturation of oxy- to deoxyhemoglobin)
  - Faint stippled or brush-like enhancement with small punctate and linear/branching vessels
  - Up to 2/3rds have enlarged collecting vein (may be mixed with venous malformation)
- Multifocal hypointensities on T2WI, GRE scans ("black dots")

Other Modality Findings
- DSA/MRA/CTA
  - Negative unless mixed malformation (e.g., venous)

Capillary Telangiectasia (CT)

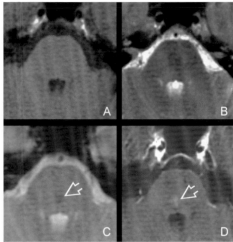

MR scans of capillary telangiectasia. The lesion is inapparent on T1- (A) and T2WI (B). The lesion (open arrows) is hypointense on T2* scan (C) and shows faint stippled, brush-like enhancement (D).

Differential Diagnosis

Metastasis
- Usually enhances strongly
- Location (gray-white junction; pons/cerebellum rare)

Cavernous Malformation
- Blood locules with fluid-fluid levels
- Abnormalities in adjacent brain (e.g., hemosiderin rim)
- Mixed capillary/cavernous or capillary venous malformation

Pathology

General
- Etiology-Pathogenesis
  - Sporadic CTs: Unknown
  - May develop as complication of radiation (usually whole brain, often for leukemia)
- Epidemiology
  - 15%-20% of all intracranial vascular malformations

Gross Pathologic or Surgical Features
- Rarely identified unless unusually large (up to 2 cm reported) or hemorrhage (from other vascular malformation) present

Microscopic Features
- Numerous dilated but histologically normal capillaries
- Normal brain between enlarged capillary channels
- Uncomplicated CTs have no gliosis, hemorrhage, Ca++
- May be histologically mixed (CM most common)
  - Blood products

Clinical Issues

Presentation
- Rarely symptomatic, usually discovered incidentally

Capillary Telangiectasia (CT)

- Rare
  - Headache
  - Vertigo, tinnitus
  - Cranial neuropathy

Natural History
- Clinically quiescent unless histologically mixed
- No change in size or configuration

Treatment & Prognosis
- None

Selected References
1. Castillo M et al: MR imaging and histologic features of capillary telangiectasia of the basal ganglia. AJNR 22: 1553-5, 2001
2. Kuker W et al: Presumed capillary telangiectasia of the pons. Eur Radiol 10: 945-50, 2000
3. Huddle DC et al: Clinically aggressive diffuse capillary telangiectasia of the brain stem. AJNR 20: 1674-7, 1999

Cavernous Malformation (CM)

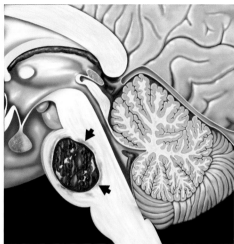

Sagittal graphic depicts typical cavernous malformation, shown here in the pons. Locules of blood with fluid-fluid levels, hemorrhage in different stages, and some flocculent Ca++ are present. Hemosiderin rim surrounds the lesion (arrows).

Key Facts
- CM (cavernous "angioma") should not be confused with cavernous **hem**angioma (true vasoproliferative neoplasm)
- CM = most common angiographically "occult" vascular malformation
- CMs exhibit range of dynamic behaviors (enlargement, regression, **de novo** formation)
- Familial CMs at high risk for hemorrhage, forming new lesions

Imaging Findings
<u>General Features</u>
- Discrete, lobulated mass
- Bleeding, variable maturation of blood products
- Best diagnostic sign = "popcorn ball" with complete hemosiderin rim

<u>CT Findings</u>
- Negative in 30%-50%
- Well-delineated round/ovoid hyperdense lesion, usually <3 cm
- Surrounding brain usually appears normal
- No mass effect unless recent hemorrhage
- Little/no enhancement

<u>MR Findings</u>
- Variable, depending on hemorrhage/stage
- Large acute hemorrhage may obscure more typical features of CM
- Reticulated "popcorn-like" lesion most typical
  - Mixed signal core, complete hemosiderin rim
  - Locules of blood with fluid-fluid levels
  - Susceptibility effect (lesion "blooms" on T2WI, T2* scans)
  - Minimal or no enhancement (may show associated VM)
- If >3 lesions, numerous punctate hypointense foci ("black dots") on GRE scans most common finding

Cavernous Malformation (CM)

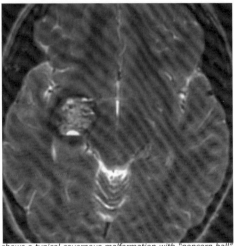

Axial T2WI shows a typical cavernous malformation with "popcorn ball" appearance (locules of blood and fluid-fluid levels) encased by a complete hemosiderin rim.

Other Modality Findings
- DSA
  - Negative ("angiographically occult vascular malformation")
    - CMs have slow intralesional flow without AV shunting
  - Avascular mass effect if large or acute hemorrhage
  - +/- Associated other malformation (e.g., VM)
  - Rare: Venous pooling, contrast "blush"

Differential Diagnosis
"Popcorn Ball" Lesion
- AVM (edema, mass effect, often single blood product)
- Hemorrhagic neoplasm (incomplete hemosiderin rim, disordered evolution of blood products, strong enhancement)
- Calcified neoplasm (e.g., oligodendroglioma; usually shows some enhancement)

Multiple "Black Dots"
- Old trauma (DAI, contusions)
- Hypertensive microbleeds (history of longstanding HTN)
- Amyloid angiopathy (elderly, demented, white matter disease)
- Capillary telangiectasias (faint brush-like enhancement)

Pathology
General
- Genetics
  - Multiple (familial) CM syndrome
    - Autosomal dominant, variable penetrance
    - Mutation in chromosomes 3,7q (KRIT1 mutation at CCM1)

Cavernous Malformation (CM)

- Etiology-Pathogenesis-Pathophysiology
  - CMs are angiogenically immature lesions with endothelial proliferation, increased neoangiogenesis
  - VEGF, βFGF, TGFα expressed;
  - Receptors (e.g., Flk-1) upregulated
- Epidemiology
  - Approximate prevalence 0.5%
  - 75% occur as solitary, sporadic lesion
  - 10%-30% multiple, familial
  - M = F

Gross Pathologic or Surgical Features
- Discrete, lobulated, bluish-purple ("mulberry-like") nodule
- Pseudocapsule of gliotic, hemosiderin-stained brain

Microscopic Features
- Thin-walled epithelial-lined spaces
- Embedded in collagenous matrix
- Hemorrhage in different stages of evolution
- +/- Ca++
- Does not contain normal brain
- May be histologically mixed (VM most common)

Clinical Issues

Presentation
- Peak presentation = 40-60y but may present in childhood
- Symptoms
  - Seizure 50%
  - Neurologic deficit 25% (may be progressive)
  - 20% asymptomatic

Natural History
- Broad range of dynamic behavior (may progress, enlarge, regress)
- **De novo** lesions may develop
- Propensity for repeated intralesional hemorrhages
  - Sporadic = .25%-.7%/year
  - Familial = approximately 1% per lesion per year
  - Risk factor for future hemorrhage = previous hemorrhage
  - Rehemorrhage rate high initially, decreases after 2-3 years

Selected References
1. Clatterbuck RE et al: The nature and fate of punctate (Type IV) cavernous malformations. Neurosurg 49: 26-32, 2001
2. Sure U et al: Endothelial proliferation, neoangiogenesis, and potential de novo generation of cerebrovascular malformations. J Neurosurg 94: 972-7, 2001
3. Brunereau L et al: Familial form of intracranial cavernous angioma. Radiol 214: 209-16, 2000

STROKE AND VASCULAR DISEASE

Acute Ischemic Stroke

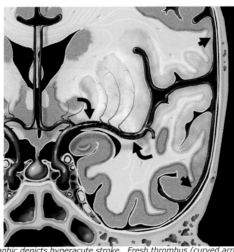

Coronal graphic depicts hyperacute stroke. Fresh thrombus (curved arrows) is seen in the proximal MCA. Retrograde flow through watershed collaterals is present (arrows). Note pallor, swelling of the basal ganglia and affected cortex with effaced G-W interfaces.

Key Facts
- "Time is brain"
- Clinical diagnosis inaccurate in 15%-20%
- Imaging diagnosis, intervention key for salvaging "at risk" tissue

Imaging Findings
General Features
- Acute thrombus in cerebral vessel(s)
- Decreased perfusion within territory of occluded vessel
- Cytotoxic edema
- Best diagnostic signs
  - CT: Hyperdense artery sign
  - MR: High signal on DWI

CT Findings (NECT)
- Hyperattenuating vessel
  - Hyperdense M1 MCA ("dense MCA sign") in 35%-50%
  - "Dot sign" = occluded MCA branches in sylvian fissure
- Loss of gray-white matter differentiation within first 3 hours
  - Subtle findings present in 50%-70% of cases
    - Lentiform nucleus obscured
    - Insular "ribbon" lost
- Parenchymal hypodensity
  - If > 1/3 MCA territory on initial CT, large lesion later
- Gyral swelling, sulcal effacement
- "Hemorrhagic transformation"
  - Delayed onset (24-48h)
  - Can be gross or petechial
  - 15%-45% of cases on NECT
  - Risk factors: Early CT signs of ischemic stroke, thromboembolic stroke, diabetes, decreased consciousness, thrombolysis

Acute Ischemic Stroke

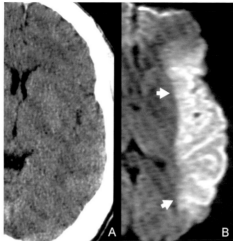

(A) NECT scan in a patient 1 hour after onset of stroke symptoms is normal. Routine MR scan was normal, but DWI disclosed acute MCA infarct (B, arrows).

MR Findings
- Conventional sequences + in 70%-80%
  - T1WI: Early cortical swelling, subtle loss of gray-white borders
  - T2WI: Hyperintensity in affected distribution
  - T1WI + contrast: Intravascular enhancement
- FLAIR
  - May be + (hyperintense) when other sequences normal
  - Intraarterial signal = early sign of major vessel occlusion

Other Modality Findings
- DSA: Vessel occlusion (cutoff, tapered, meniscus, tram track), slow antegrade flow, retrograde collateral flow across watershed
- Triphasic perfusion CTA: Ischemic core, penumbra depicted
- TCD: Proximal occlusion in 70% of thrombolysis-eligible patients
- DWI: Restricted diffusion (high signal), improves accuracy to 95%
- ADC: Intermediate ("at risk" tissue) to significantly reduced (brain that will infarct); evolves faster for thromboembolic vs. watershed infarct
- Bolus-tracking PWI with rCBF map: Decreased perfusion (75% are larger than lesion on DWI, shows ischemic "at risk" tissue)

Imaging Recommendations
- NECT scan to detect hemorrhage (e.g., HTN-related bleed)
- MRI (with FLAIR, DWI +/- PWI)
- DSA with thrombolysis in selected patients

Differential Diagnosis
Hyperdense Vessel Sign
- Normal (circulating blood is slightly hyperdense to brain)
- High hematocrit
- Microcalcification in vessel wall
- Low density brain (e.g., diffuse cerebral edema) makes vessels appear relatively hyperdense

Acute Ischemic Stroke

Parenchymal Hypodensity
- Infiltrating neoplasm
- Inflammation (e.g., encephalitis)

Pathology
General
- Etiology-Pathogenesis-Pathophysiology
  - Early: Critical disturbance in CBF
    - Severely ischemic core has CBF <6 cm^3/100g^{-1}/min^{-1}
    - Causes oxygen depletion, energy failure, terminal depolarization, ion homeostasis failure
    - Represents bulk of final infarct
    - Ischemic penumbra CBF between 7 and 20 cm^3/100g^{-1}/min^{-1}
  - Secondary changes include excitotoxicity, SD-like depolarizations, disturbance of ion homeostasis
  - Evolution from ischemia to infarction depends on many factors (e.g., BP fluctuations, embolic fragmentation, reperfusion)
  - Delayed effects: Inflammation, apoptosis
- Epidemiology
  - Second most common worldwide cause of death
  - Major cause of long-term disability

Gross Pathologic or Surgical Features
- Acute thrombosis of major vessel
- Pale, swollen brain; GM/WM boundaries "smudged"

Microscopic Features
- After 4h: Eosinophilic neurons with pyknotic nuclei
- 15-24h: Neutrophils invade; necrotic nuclei look like "eosionophilic ghosts"
- 2-3 days: Blood-derived phagocytes
- 1 week: Reactive astrocytosis, increased capillary density
- End result: Fluid-filled cavity lined by astrocytes

Clinical Issues
Presentation
- Varies with vascular distribution

Natural History
- "Malignant" MCA infarct (coma, death)
  - Up to 10% of all stroke patients
  - Fatal brain swelling with increased intracranial pressure

Treatment & Prognosis
- Generally unfavorable outcome without treatment
- Patient selection = most important factor in treatment outcome
  - < 6h
  - CT shows no parenchymal hematoma
  - < 1/3 MCA territory hypodensity

Selected References
1. Parsons MW et al: Perfusion MRI maps in hyperacute stroke. Stroke 32: 1581-7, 2001
2. Huang I-J et al: Time course of cerebral infarction in the middle cerebral artery territory: Deep watershed versus territorial subtypes on diffusion-weighted MR images. Radiol 221: 35-42, 2001
3. Gaskill-Shipley MF: Routine CT evaluation of acute stroke. Neuroimag Clin N Amer 9: 411-22, 1999

Pediatric/Young Adult Stroke

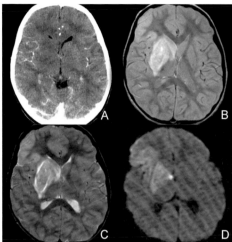

Child with acute chickenpox vasculitis. (A) CECT scan shows loss of the interface between the right basal ganglia and surrounding white matter. Axial PD- (B) and T2WI (C) show high signal in the basal ganglia/internal/external capsule as well as the right posterior frontal cortex. (D) DWI shows restriction.

Key Facts
- Pediatric stroke etiologies extremely varied
- Neonate/infant: R-L cardiac shunt, birth trauma
- <15 y: Prothrombotic states cause 20-50% of arterial ischemic strokes, 33-99% sinovenous thrombosis
- >15 y: Dissection, atherothrombosis, more "traditional" risk factors

Imaging Findings
General Features
- Similar to adults (see "Acute Stroke")

CT Findings
- Similar to adults (see "Acute Stroke")
- Look for clues to stroke etiology
  - Basal ganglia Ca++ (MELAS, cranial irradiation)
  - Vascular anomaly (check presence/size of carotid canal)
  - Pre-existing atrophy (SLE, other collagen-vascular)
  - Enhancing "dots" in basal ganglia ("moyamoya" collaterals)

MR Findings
- Similar to adults (see "Acute Stroke")
- Look for clues to stroke etiology
  - Stigmata of neurocutaneous disorder (e.g., NF-1)
  - Midline malformations
  - Metabolic disease (e.g., Melas, Leigh)

Other Modality Findings
- DWI: Acute restriction + chronic changes (new stroke superimposed on old, e.g., sickle-cell, moyamoya)

Imaging Recommendations
- Screening CECT may give early clue to
  - Perfusion of normal vs. "drop out" of ischemic tissue

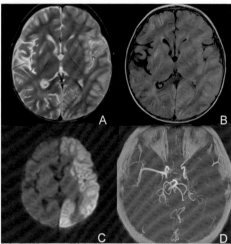

Axial T2WI (A), FLAIR scans (B) in idiopathic progressive arteriopathy of childhood show right hemisphere atrophy, basal ganglia lacunes, left cortical edema. (C) DWI shows restriction. (D) MRA shows occluded left supraclinoid ICA with basal ("moyamoya") collaterals.

- o Circle of Willis patency
- o Presence of sinovenous occlusion
- MR/MRA/MRV
- DWI

Differential Diagnosis
Nonischemic Causes of Acute Childhood Hemiparesis
- Todd's paresis
- A.D.E.M.

"Newly Noticed" Hemiparesis
- Perinatal infarct
- Congenital anomaly (i.e., schizencephaly)
- Caution
  - o Hemiparesis sometimes noticed only when child old enough to walk/use hands purposefully
  - o Brain anomaly/perinatal stroke may seem "acute" at 9 to 18 mo

Pathology
General
- Etiology-Pathogenesis-Pathophysiology (multifactorial)
  - o Cardiac (embolism, valve anomaly, left atrial myxoma)
  - o Congenital prothrombotic disorders
    - ▪ Resistance to: Activated protein C
    - ▪ Deficiencies of: Antithrombin, protein S or C
    - ▪ Presence of: Factor V-Leiden, anti-cardiolipin/anti-phospholipid antibodies, lupus anticoagulant, etc.
  - o Acquired prothrombotic disorders
    - ▪ Hyperlipidemia, polycythemia, iron deficiency anemia, platelet disorders, leukemia, chemotherapy-related

- o Other inherited disorders
  - ▪ Skull base anomaly with absent carotid canal (e.g., Morning-glory syndrome with colobomas, vasculopathy, pituitary malfunction, sphenopharyngeal encephalocele)
  - ▪ Neurocutaneous syndrome: NF-1, TS
  - ▪ Vasculopathies: CADASIL, CARASIL, sickle-cell anemia
  - ▪ Metabolic: MELAS, homocysteinuria, premature aging (progeria)
- o Other acquired disorders
  - ▪ Migraine, dissection
  - ▪ Non-accidental injury
  - ▪ Vasculopathies: Chickenpox; isolated CNS angiitis; systemic angiitis (Kawasaki, Takayasu, polyarteritis nodosa, Behçet's); moyamoya phenomenon (idiopathic or secondary)
  - ▪ Any progressive vasculopathy ⇒ moyamoya-like radiology
  - ▪ Teen/young adult: Add "street" drugs, oral contraceptives
  - ▪ Young adult: Add atheroembolic, cigarette smoking, diabetes

Staging or Grading Criteria
- Moyamoya 1-6
  - o 1 = stenosis distal ICA
  - o 2-5 = opening then closing of basal collaterals
  - o 6= dependence on transdural collaterals

Clinical Issues
Presentation
- Infant
  - o Seizure
  - o Poor feeding, developmental delay
- Older children: Depends upon size, vascular distribution

Treatment & Prognosis
- Treat etiologic factor(s)
- Anticoagulation (aspirin/heparin/Coumadin)
- Immunosuppression (autoimmune)
- Symptomatic moyamoya (synangiosis?)

Selected References
1. Chan AK, deVeber G. Prothrombotic disorders and ischemic stroke in children. Semin Pediatr Neurol 7: 301-8, 2000
2. Williams LS et al: Subtypes of ischemic stroke in children and young adults. Neurology 49: 1541-5, 1997
3. Giroud M et al: Stroke in children under 16 years of age. Clinical and etiological difference with adults. Acta Neurol Scand 96: 401-6, 1997

Primary Hemorrhage (pICH)

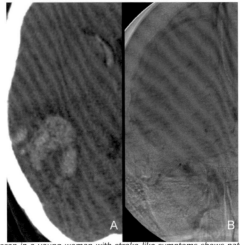

(A) NECT scan in a young woman with stroke-like symptoms shows patchy parietal cortical/subcortical hemorrhage. (B) DSA, anteroposterior view, venous phase, shows the right TS is occluded. Venous infarct.

Key Facts
- Nontraumatic pICH causes 15%-20% of acute "strokes"
- Hypertension (HTN), cerebral amyloid angiopathy (CAA), coagulopathy most common causes of pICH in elderly
- Patients< 45y often have underlying vascular lesion such as aneurysm, cerebral vascular malformation (CVM), venous occlusion

Imaging Findings
General Features
- Best diagnostic signs
  - Deep (ganglionic) hematoma in HTN
  - Lobar/subcortical hematoma in CAA, CVM, venous occlusion
CT Findings
- Round/elliptical parenchymal mass
  - Acute ICH usually hyperdense
  - May be mixed iso-/hyperdense if rapid bleeding, coagulopathy
  - Peripheral low density (edema)
- Ganglionic ICH may extend into lateral ventricle
MR Findings
- Signal intensity varies with numerous factors including
  - Pulse sequence
  - Flip angle
  - Susceptibility effects (Hgb deoxygenation)
  - RBC status (lysed or intact)
- Hyperacute hematoma (<6h)
  - Center (oxygenated hematoma): Iso-/hyperintense, heterogeneous on T2-, T2*
  - Periphery (deoxygenated Hgb, clot-tissue interface): Hypointense on T2-, T2*
  - Rim (vasogenic edema): Hypointense on T1-, hyper on T2WI
- +/- Evidence of previous hemorrhage in other areas

Primary Hemorrhage (pICH)

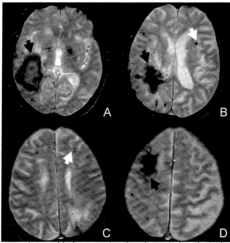

(A-D) GRE scans in an elderly normotensive demented patient show two lobar hemorrhages (black arrows), multiple small "black dots" elsewhere (white arrows). Extensive white matter disease is present. Amyloid angiopathy.

    o   Low signal intensity foci on T2* in up to 1/3 of cases

<u>Other Modality Findings</u>
- DWI: Hypo- or mixed hypo/hyperintense (early hematoma)
- ADC: Markedly reduced (early hematoma)
- DSA: May not demonstrate vascular malformation in acute stage
- PET: May be useful for neoplastic vs. nonneoplastic hematoma

<u>Imaging Recommendations</u>
- NECT: If hematoma/history typical for HTN, stop
- If atypical hematoma or unclear history, do contrast-enhanced MR (with GRE for co-existing microhemorrhage)
- DSA if suspicious for thrombosed CVM

Differential Diagnosis
<u>HTN vs. CAA (see "Cerebral Amyloid Angiopathy")</u>
- Both occur in older patients
- Both may have evidence for previous hemorrhages
- HTN usually ganglionic; amyloid usually lobar
- Amyloid usually >70y, normotensive, demented

<u>Hypertensive Bleed vs. Neoplasm, Vascular Malformation</u>
- HTN unusual in young patients unless drug abuse (e.g., cocaine)
- Neoplasm often has disordered evolution of hemorrhage, foci of contrast enhancement

<u>Cortical Vein Thrombosis</u>
- Adjacent dural sinus often (but not always!) thrombosed

Pathology
<u>General</u>
- Etiology-Pathogenesis-Pathophysiology
  - o   Older patients
    - Basal ganglionic = HTN
    - Lobar = amyloid angiopathy

Primary Hemorrhage (pICH)

- Neoplasm (2%-14% of "spontaneous" ICH)
- Coagulopathy
- Venous occlusion, vascular malformation, aneurysm
  o Younger patients
    - Lobar = CVM
    - Other: Drug use, vasculitis, venous thrombosis
- Epidemiology
  o 15%-20% of acute "strokes"

Gross Pathologic, Surgical Features
- Acute ganglionic/lobar hematoma

Microscopic Features
- Co-existing microangiopathy common in amyloid, HTN

Staging or Grading Criteria
- Clinical ICH score correlates with 30-day mortality
  o Admission GCS
  o Age >80y, ICH volume
  o Infratentorial
  o Presence of IVH

Clinical Issues

Presentation
- > 50% of patients with pICH do not have HTN
- 90% of patients with recurrent pICH are hypertensive

Natural History
- Hematoma enlargement common in first 24-48h
  o Risk factors = EtOH, low fibrinogen, coagulopathy, irregularly shaped hematoma, disturbed consciousness
- 30% of patients rebleed within 1 year

Treatment & Prognosis
- Mortality 30%-55% in first month
- Surgical evacuation controversial
- Recovery poor; most survivors have significant deficits

Selected References
1. Wiesmann M et al: Detection of hyperacute parenchymal hemorrhage of the brain using echo-planar T2*-weighted and diffusion-weighted MRI. Eur. Radiol 11: 849-53, 2001
2. Linfante I et al: MRI features of intracerebral hemorrhage within 2 hours from symptom onset. Stroke 30: 2263-7, 1999
3. Offenbacher H et al: MR of cerebral abnormalities concomitant with primary intracerebral hematomas. JNR 17: 573-8, 1996

Hypertensive Hemorrhage (hICH)

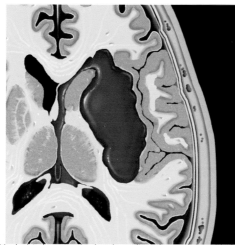

Axial graphic depicts hypertensive basal ganglionic hemorrhage with dissection into the lateral ventricle. Hematoma epicenter is lateral putamen/ external capsule.

Key Facts
- HTN most common cause of spontaneous ICH between 45-70 years
- Ganglionic bleed is most common pattern
- Chronic HTN may cause multifocal "black dots" on T2WI, T2* scans

Imaging Findings
General Features
- Two distinct patterns seen with hypertensive hemorrhage
  - Acute focal hematoma
  - Multiple subacute/chronic "microbleeds"
  - Best diagnostic sign= putamen hematoma in patient with HTN
CT Findings
- Elliptical high density mass
  - Most common = between putamen, insular cortex
  - Other sites = thalamus, brainstem
- Mixed density if coagulopathy, active bleeding
- Other: Hydrocephalus, IVH, herniation
MR Findings
- See "Primary ICH"
- Contrast extravasation = active hemorrhage, growing hematoma
- Multifocal hypointense lesions on T2*
  - Common with longstanding HTN
  - Also seen with amyloid angiopathy
Other Modality Findings
- DSA/CTA
  - Almost always normal if HTN + deep ganglionic hemorrhage
  - May show avascular mass effect
Imaging Recommendations
- NECT scan
- If older patient with HTN, typical hematoma, stop

Hypertensive Hemorrhage (hICH)

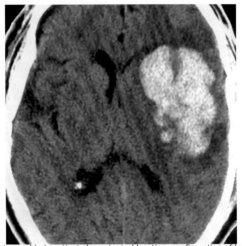

NECT scan in an elderly patient shows typical location, configuration of hypertensive ICH. Blood pressure was 180/120.

- If no clear cause of hemorrhage or atypical appearance, consider MR (include contrast-enhanced, T2* sequences) + MRA
- If MR shows co-existing multifocal "black dots," stop
- If MR shows atypical hematoma, CTA
- If CTA inconclusive, consider DSA

Differential Diagnosis

Basal Ganglionic Hemorrhage
- Vascular malformation (younger patients)
- Hemorrhagic neoplasm (often mixed signal, enhancing)
- Other: Coagulopathy, drug abuse

Lobar Hemorrhage
- Amyloid angiopathy (elderly, demented, normotensive; rarely involves deep subcortical nuclei)
- Thrombosed AVM or dAVS (younger patients with stagnating vessels, early draining veins on angiography)
- Cortical vein thrombosis (co-existing dural sinus thrombosis often-but not always-present)

Multifocal "Black Dots"
- Hemorrhagic DAI
- Multiple cavernous/capillary malformations
- Amyloid angiopathy

Pathology

General
- General Path Comments (location)
    o Striatocapsular (putamen/external capsule) 60%-65%
    o Thalamus 15%-25%
    o Pons, cerebellum 10%
    o Lobar 5%-15%
    o Multifocal "microbleeds" 1%-5%

Hypertensive Hemorrhage (hICH)

- Etiology-Pathogenesis
  - "Bleeding globe" (penetrating artery aneurysm)
  - Chronic HTN with atherosclerosis, fibrinoid necrosis, abrupt wall rupture +/- pseudoaneurysm formation
  - N.B.: 10%-15% of hypertensive patients with spontaneous ICH have underlying aneurysm or AVM
- Epidemiology
  - 50% of primary ICHs caused by hypertensive hemorrhage

Gross Pathologic or Surgical Features
- Large ganglionic hematoma +/- IVH
- Subfalcine herniation, hydrocephalus common
- Co-existing small chronic hemorrhages, ischemic lesions common

Microscopic Features
- Fibrous balls (fibrosed miliary aneurysm)
- Severe arteriosclerosis with hyalinization, pseudoaneurysm (lacks media/IEL)

Clinical Issues

Presentation
- Large ICHs present with sensorimotor deficits, impaired consciousness
- Seasonal, diurnal blood pressure variations cause higher incidence of ICH in colder months

Natural History
- Bleeding can persist for up to 6h following ictus
- Neurologic deterioration common within 48h
  - Increasing hematoma
  - Edema
  - Development of hydrocephalus
  - Herniation syndromes
- Recurrent hICH in 5%-10% of cases, usually different location

Treatment & Prognosis
- Prognosis related to location, size of ICH
- 80% mortality in massive ICH with IVH
- One-third of survivors are severely disabled
- Stereotaxic evacuation may improve outcome

Selected References
1. Chung C-S et al: Striatocapsular haemorrhage. Brain 123: 1850-62, 2000
2. Broderick JP et al: Guidelines for the management of spontaneous intracerebral hemorrhage. Stroke 30: 905-15, 1999
3. Tanaka A et al: Small chronic hemorrhages and ischemic lesions in association with spontaneous intracerebral hematomas. Stroke 30: 1637-42, 1999

Hypertensive Encephalopathy

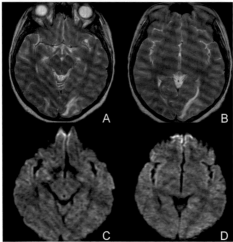

(A, B) Axial T2WI in a patient with acute severe HTN shows subcortical high-signal intensity in both occipital poles (left > right). (C, D) DWI shows no restriction, indicating no ischemia is present. The lesions resolved with BP normalization.

Key Facts
- Synonyms = posterior reversible encephalopathy syndrome (PRES), reversible posterior leukoencephalopathy syndrome (RPLS)
- Diverse causes (severe HTN, immunosuppressive agents, etc.)
- Etiology = breakthrough of autoregulation with BBB disruption, vasogenic edema
- Typically reversible with blood pressure normalization

Imaging Findings
General Features
- Cortical/subcortical edema with predilection for posterior circulation (parietal, occipital lobes)
- Best diagnostic sign= Patient with acute HTN, patchy lesions in PCA territory

CT Findings
- NECT: Bilateral symmetric hypodense areas in posterior parietal, occipital lobes, sometimes basal ganglia
- CECT: May have mild patchy/punctate enhancement

MR Findings
- Cortical/subcortical lesions (hypo- on T1WI, hyperintense on T2WI)
- FLAIR
  - Cortical lesions in 95% (high signal intensity)
  - +/- Symmetric lesions in basal ganglia
- Complicated/severe cases may have petechial hemorrhages, patchy enhancement
- Less common
  - Extensive brain stem hyperintensity
  - Generalized white matter edema

Hypertensive Encephalopathy

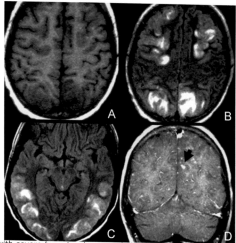

A patient with severe hypertensive encephalopathy shows striking abnormalities in the vascular watershed zones and PCA territories. (A) T1WI, (B, C) FLAIR, and post-contrast coronal T1WI are shown. Note patchy enhancement (D, arrow).

Other Modality Findings
- DWI: Usually isointense with normal WM (can occasionally be hypointense)
- ADC: Markedly elevated

Imaging Recommendations
- Contrast-enhanced MR+ DWI
- Repeat scan after BF normalized

Differential Diagnosis
Acute Cerebral Ischemia
- Clinical history (HTN, time of symptom onset) important
- DWI usually high signal

Transient Cerebral Hyperemia
- Ictal/postictal
- Rapid decompression of chronic SDH
- Postcarotid endarterectomy hyperperfusion syndrome

Pontine Encephalopathy (Pontine Reversible Edema)
- Pontine glioma
- Brainstem ischemia/infarction

In Setting of Immunosuppression, RPLS vs
- Progressive multifocal leukoencephalopathy
- Demyelinating disease
- Gliomatosis cerebri

Pathology
General
- Etiology-Pathogenesis-Pathophysiology
  - Combination of acute HTN + endothelial damage
  - **Not** cytotoxic edema (ischemia/infarction rare)
  - **Is** "autoregulatory overload" with vasogenic edema
    - Arteriolar dilatation with cerebral hyperperfusion

- Hydrostatic leakage (extravasation, transudation of fluid and macromolecules through arteriolar, capillary walls)
- Interstitial fluid accumulates in cortex, subcortical white matter
- Posterior circulation sparsely innervated by sympathetic nerves (predilection for parietal, occipital lobes)
  - Specific causes
    - Eclampsia/preeclampsia
    - Severe HTN
    - Cyclosporine toxicity
    - Uremic encephalopathies

Gross Pathologic or Surgical Features
- Common
  - Cortical/subcortical edema
  - +/- Petechial hemorrhage in parietal, occipital lobes
- Less common: Lesions in basal ganglia, cerebellum, brain stem, anterior frontal lobes

Microscopic Features
- Usually no residual abnormalities after HTN corrected
- Autopsy in severe cases shows microvascular fibrinoid necrosis and ischemic microinfarcts
- Chronic HTN associated with mural thickening, deposition of collagen, laminin, fibronectin in cerebral arterioles

Clinical Issues
Presentation
- Headache, nausea, vomiting, seizures, visual disturbances, altered mental status
- Acute or subacute systemic hypertension
- **Some patients, especially children, may even be normotensive or have minimally elevated BP!**

Natural History
- May be life-threatening
- Most cases resolve completely with blood pressure normalization
- Permanent infarction rare

Treatment & Prognosis
- Favorable outcome with prompt recognition, treatment of HTN

Selected References
1. Mukherjee P et al: Reversible posterior leukoencephalopathy syndrome: Evaluation with diffusion-tensor MR imaging. Radiol 219: 756-65, 2001
2. Provenzale JM et al: Quantitative assessment of diffusion abnormalities in posterior reversible encephalopathy syndrome. AJNR 22: 1455-61, 2001
3. Port JD et al: Reversible intracerebral pathologic entities mediated by vascular autoregulatory dysfunction. Radiographics 18: 353-67, 1998

Hypoxic Ischemic (HIE)

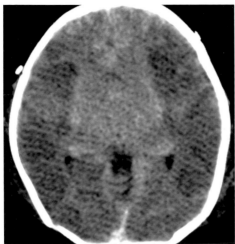

NECT scan in a newborn with acute partial asphyxia shows bilateral diffuse cortical/ subcortical low density with relative preservation of the basal ganglia and thalami.

Key Facts
- Findings differ with
  - Gestational age, maturity of cerebral vasculature
  - Chronic vs. acute ischemia
  - Partial (usual) vs. profound (uncommon) hypoxia

Imaging Findings
General Features
- Partial ischemia (mild/moderate reduced CBF)
  - Primarily cortical/subcortical (parasagittal "border zone")
  - Basal ganglia, brainstem/cerebellum relatively spared
- Profound ischemia (severely decreased or no CBF)
  - Affects areas of high metabolic demand
  - Basal ganglia (globus pallidus, posterior putamen, lateral thalamus)
  - Myelinated or actively myelinating white matter
  - Perirolandic cortex (at depths of sulci)
- Best diagnostic sign = deep GM/WM interfaces lost (profound ischemia)
CT Findings
- Partial ischemia
  - Acute
    - Loss of cortical, insular "ribbon"
    - Cortex/subcortical WM edema
  - Chronic
    - Ulegyria (border zone volume loss), diffuse atrophy
- Profound ischemia
  - Acute
    - Low density basal ganglia, loss of GM/WM interfaces
    - +/- Petechial hemorrhages
  - Chronic
    - Atrophic basal ganglia, thalami; +/- hazy Ca++
    - +/- Slit-like lacunes

Hypoxic Ischemic (HIE)

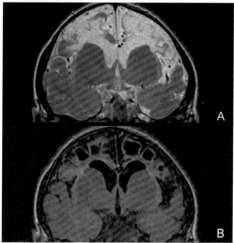

Follow-up coronal T2WI (A) and FLAIR scans (B) in a child who suffered partial ischemia at birth show striking encephalomalacia with ulegyria in both parasagittal watershed zones. Note the basal ganglia are spared.

MR Findings
- Partial ischemia
  - Hyperintense cortex/subcortical WM on T2WI, FLAIR
- Profound
  - Bright T1 more pronounced than bright T2 (ventrolateral thalamus, globus pallidus, perirolandic cortex, etc.)
  - >37weeks, T1 signal loss (myelinated posterior limb IC)

Other Modality Findings
- Sonography: Useful in premature, much less in full term infant
- DWI
  - Neonate has mostly unmyelinated ("wet") brain
  - Acute ischemia (1-7 days) shows restriction
- MRS
  - Lactate normal feature of developing brain <37 weeks gestation but decreases as normal finding >37 weeks
  - Presence of α-glutamate/glutamine peaks correlates with moderate to severe injury
  - NAA low for age correlates with poor prognosis

Imaging Recommendations
- DWI (most sensitive in early imaging of acute ischemia)
- Standard MR may take 72 hours to depict maximal damage
- CT may take up to 4 days (follow-up at 2 weeks recommended)

Differential Diagnosis

Kernicterus
- Can mimic profound injury on acute T1WI but lacks abnormal thalamic signal, clinical/laboratory evidence of hyperbilirubinemia
- Can be accentuated by sepsis, hypoxia

Hypoxic Ischemic (HIE)

Metabolic Disorder
- Inherited
  - o Mitochondrial encephalopathy, urea cycle disorders
- Acquired
  - o Neonatal hypoglycemia "attacks" parietal/occipital lobes
  - o Manganese toxicity mimics T1 basal ganglia changes of HIE

Pathology
General
- General Path Comments
  - o Ischemia often multi-organ (e.g., cardiac, renal)
- Embryology
  - o Vascular watershed ("border zone") shifts from periventricular in premature to parasagittal (term) infant
  - o Premature: Reduced perfusion of periventricular WM (site of oligodendrocyte proliferation for myelination) causes PVL
- Etiology-Pathogenesis-Pathophysiology
  - o Partial ischemia: CBF shifts to basal ganglia/brainstem/cerebellum
  - o Profound: No time to shift CBF
    - ▪ Highest metabolic demand/actively myelinating regions affected
  - o Different patterns of asphyxia seen at different gestational ages
    - ▪ Glutamate released into synaptic clefts, NMDA receptors
    - ▪ Cascade of reactions in postsynaptic neurons leads to cell death
    - ▪ Postsynaptic receptor distribution changes with development, gives different damage patterns at different gestational ages
- Epidemiology
  - o Up to 2/1000 (0.2%) live births

Gross Pathologic, Surgical Features
- Parasagittal ulegyria (chronic partial)
- Hippocampal, basal ganglia atrophy (profound)

Microscopic Features
- <30 gestational weeks: Liquefaction, resorption of parenchyma
- >30 weeks: Reactive astrogliosis, macrophages

Clinical Issues
Presentation
- Sarnat stages of HIE encephalopathy
  - o I (mild): Hyperalert/irritable, mydriasis, EEG normal
  - o II (moderate): Lethargy, hypotonia, decreased HR, seizures
  - o III (severe): Stupor, flaccid, reflexes absent; seizures

Natural History
- Varies from normal outcome (Sarnat I) to spastic quadriparesis, developmental delay, microcephaly, seizures (Sarnat III)
- Choreoathetosis after 1 year common in survivors of profound asphyxia

Treatment & Prognosis
- Correct hypoxia, metabolic disturbances (hypoglycemia, acidosis)

Selected References
1. Bydder GM et al: Diffusion-weighted imaging in neonates. Childs Nerv Syst 17: 190-4, 2001
2. Barkovich AJ et al: Prediction of neuromotor outcome in perinatal asphyxia: Evaluation of MR scoring systems. AJNR 19: 143-9, 1998
3. Azzarelli B et al: Hypoxic-ischemic encephalopathy in areas of primary myelination: A neuroimaging and PET study. Pediatr Neurol 14: 108-16, 1996

Venous Occlusion

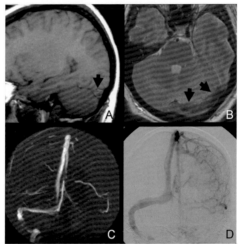

Acute TS thrombosis. Clot is isointense with brain on T1WI (A, arrow), hypointense on T2WI (B, arrows). MRV and DSA show occluded left TS (C, D).

Key Facts
- 1% of acute strokes
- Clinical diagnosis often elusive
- Early imaging findings may be subtle, often overlooked

Imaging Findings
General Features
- Thrombus in dural sinus, vein(s)
- Parenchymal edema, petechial hemorrhages
- Best diagnostic sign = "empty delta" on CECT, contrast-enhanced MR
CT Findings
- NECT
  - Hyperdense dural sinus > cortical vein ("cord sign")
  - +/- Parenchymal abnormality
    - Cortical/subcortical petechial hemorrhages, edema
    - If ICVs occlude, thalami/basal ganglia are hypodense
- CECT
  - "Empty delta" sign (enhancing dura surrounds nonenhancing thrombus) in 25%-30% of cases
  - "Shaggy," irregular veins (collateral channels)
MR Findings
- Signal varies with age of clot
  - Acute
    - Absent "flow void"
    - Clot iso- on T1, hypointense on T2WI
  - Subacute: Hyperintense on T1-, T2WI
- Venous infarct (50% of cases)
  - Gyral swelling, sulcal effacement
    - Hyperintense (T2WI, FLAIR)
    - Petechial hemorrhage (cortical/subcortical)
  - Patchy enhancement

Venous Occlusion

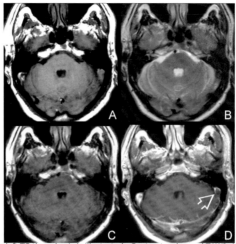

(A-D) Acute left TS thrombosis is illustrated. Contrast-enhanced T1WI shows "empty delta sign" (D, arrow), caused by enhancing dura surrounding nonenhancing clot.

Other Modality Findings
- MRV/CTV
  - Loss of vascular flow signal
  - "Frayed" or "shaggy" appearance of venous sinus
  - Abnormal collateral channels (e.g., enlarged medullary veins)
- DWI/ADC imaging findings variable, heterogeneous
- SPECT/PET: Decreased rCBF

Imaging Recommendations
- NECT, CECT scans +/- CTV
- If CT scan negative, MRI with MRV
- If MRV equivocal, DSA

Differential Diagnosis

Normal
- Blood in vessels normally slightly hyperdense on NECT scans

Anatomic Variant
- Congenital hypoplastic/absent transverse sinus
- "High-splitting" tentorium

"Giant" Arachnoid Granulation
- Round/ovoid filling defect (clot is long, linear)
- CSF density/signal intensity

False "Empty Delta" Sign
- SDH, SDE

Neoplasm
- Venous infarct can enhance, mimic neoplasm

Pathology

General
- Genetics (inherited predisposing conditions)
  - Resistance to activated protein C (typically due to factor V Leiden mutation) = most common cause of sporadic CVT

Venous Occlusion

- o   Protein S deficiency
- o   Prothrombin (factor II) gene mutation (G20210A)
- Etiology-Pathogenesis-Pathophysiology
  - o   Wide spectrum of causes (>100 identified)
    - ▪ Trauma, infection, inflammation
    - ▪ Pregnancy, oral contraceptives
    - ▪ Metabolic (dehydration, thyrotoxicosis, cirrhosis, etc.)
    - ▪ Hematological (coagulopathy)
    - ▪ Collagen-vascular disorders (e.g., APLA syndrome)
    - ▪ Vasculitis (e.g., Behcet)
  - o   Most common pattern: Thrombus initially forms in dural sinus
    - ▪ Clot propagates into cortical veins
    - ▪ Venous drainage obstructed, venous pressure elevated
    - ▪ BBB breakdown with vasogenic edema, hemorrhage
    - ▪ Venous infarct with cytotoxic edema ensues
- Epidemiology
  - o   1% of acute strokes

Gross Pathologic or Surgical Features
- Sinus occluded, distended by acute clot
- Thrombus in adjacent cortical veins
- Adjacent cortex edematous, usually with petechial hemorrhage

Staging or Grading Criteria
- Venous ischemia
  - o   Type 1: No abnormality
  - o   Type 2: High signal on T2WI/FLAIR; no enhancement
  - o   Type 3: High signal on T2WI/FLAIR; enhancement present
  - o   Type 4: Hemorrhage or venous infarction

Clinical Issues
Presentation
- Extremely variable (from asymptomatic to coma, death)
- Common: Headache, nausea, vomiting +/- neurologic deficit

Natural History
- Up to 50% of cases progress to venous infarction
- Potentially fatal

Treatment & Prognosis
- Heparin +/- rtPA
- Endovascular thrombolysis

Selected References
1.   Liang L et al: Evaluation of the intracranial dural sinuses with a 3D contrast-enhanced MP-RAGE sequence. AJNR 22: 481-92, 2001
2.   Kawaguchi T et al: Classification of venous ischemia with MRI. J Clin Neurosci 8 (suppl 1): 82-88, 2001
3.   Provenzale JM et al: Dural sinus thrombosis: Findings on CT and MR imaging and diagnostic pitfalls. AJR 170: 777-83, 1998

Atherosclerosis (ASVD)

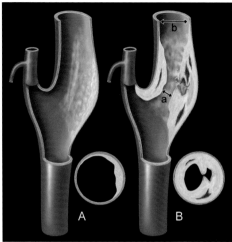

Graphic depiction of mild and severe carotid atherosclerosis (ASVD). (A) Earliest signs of ASVD are "fatty streaks" and slight intimal thickening. (B) Severe stenosis with intraplaque hemorrhage, ulceration and platelet emboli are shown. NASCET calculation % stenosis= b-a/b x 100

Key Facts
- Atherogenesis is a complex, multifactorial process
- Carotid bifurcation is most common site in head, neck
- Spectrum of pathology includes ectasia, stenosis, ulceration with platelet thrombi, embolization + silent or symptomatic infarction

Imaging Findings
General Features
- Best diagnostic sign= smooth or irregular narrowing of proximal ICA

CT Findings
- Ca++ in vessel wall (ICA, BA most common sites)
- Ectasia, tortuosity
- Fusiform dilatation
- Stenosis, occlusion (CTA)

MR Findings
- Lumen narrowed, wall thickened
- Absent "flow void" (occurs with occlusion, very slow flow)
- Stenosis (severe narrowing causes "flow gap" on MRA)

Other Modality Findings
- U/S
  - Plaque characteristics and clinical correlation
    - Hypoechoic plaques are independent risk factor for stroke
    - Acoustic shadowing correlates with ischemic stroke
  - Increased intima/media thickness = sign of early ASVD but clinical significance controversial
- DSA
  - Plaque surface irregularity associated with increased stroke risk at all degrees of stenosis
  - Detects "tandem" (siphon) stenoses, depicts collateral circulation

Atherosclerosis (ASVD)

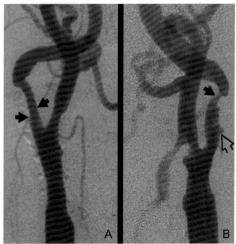

Two patients with carotid ASVD. (A) Smooth calcified plaque is present at the distal common, proximal internal carotid artery (arrows). (B) High-grade stenosis (black arrow) with irregularities (open arrow) is present. This patient had TIAs.

- [111]In Platelet Scintigraphy
  - o Detects thrombotic complications in carotid plaque

Imaging Recommendations
- U/S as initial screening procedure
- CTA/MRA
- Consider DSA prior to endarterectomy

Differential Diagnosis

Dissection
- Spares bulb
- Usually smoother, longer narrowing
- No Ca++

Pathology

General
- General Path Comments
  - o Severity of vessel narrowing is important
  - o Plaque instability, rupture, local thrombus, potential for distal (artery-to-artery) embolization also important
- Genetics
  - o Probably multigenic
  - o Many specific polymorphisms identified
- Etiology-Pathogenesis-Pathophysiology
  - o ASVD development, progression is complex, multifactorial
    - Diet, genes
    - Mechanical factors (e.g., anatomic variations, wall shear stress)
    - Role of infection (e.g., Helicobacter, Chlamydia), inflammation (activated endothelial cells, cytokine release) controversial

Atherosclerosis (ASVD)

- Epidemiology
- Leading cause of morbidity, mortality in Western world
  - Ischemic stroke accounts for up to 40% of deaths in elderly
  - Cerebral infarcts occur in >70% of patients with carotid occlusion
  - 90% of large, recent cerebral infarcts caused by thromboemboli
  - Lacunar infarcts correlate with both HTN, ASVD

Gross Pathologic or Surgical Features
- Intimal "fatty streaks" early sign
- As disease progresses, fibrotic cap covers core of foam cells, necrotic debris, cholesterol

Microscopic Features
- Monocyte-derived macrophages, smooth muscle cells proliferate
- Become lipid-filled "foam cells"
- Neovascularity may cause intraplaque hemorrhage
- Ulceration may ensue, platelet adhesion/thrombi form

Staging or Grading Criteria
- See "Carotid Stenosis"

Clinical Issues
Presentation
- Variable
  - Can be asymptomatic
  - Bruit
  - Stroke
- Risk (stroke) increases with smoking, HTN, diabetes, overweight, inferior socioeconomic circumstances

Natural History
- Progressive; significant stenosis may cause decreased perfusion
- Artery-to-artery emboli

Treatment & Prognosis
- Endarterectomy if carotid stenosis = or > 70%

Selected References
1. Ameriso SF et al: Detection of Helicobacter pylori in human carotid atherosclerotic plaques. Stroke 32: 385-91, 2001
2. Shaaban AM, Duerinckx AJ: Wall shear stress and early atherosclerosis: A review. AJR 174: 1657-65, 2000
3. Ballotta E et al: Carotid plaque gross morphology and clinical presentation: A prospective study of 457 carotid artery specimens. J Surg Res 89: 78-84, 2000

Carotid Stenosis

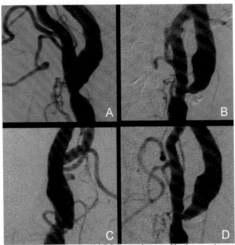

(A-D). 4 views of a common carotid DSA are shown. Maximum stenosis is profiled in B. For calculation of % stenosis, see graphic for atherosclerosis.

Key Facts
- Stroke is second most common worldwide cause of death
- Most cerebral infarcts occur in carotid vascular territory
- Carotid stenosis =/> 70% associated with significant stroke risk, benefit from endarterectomy

Imaging Findings
General Features
- Smooth or irregular narrowing of internal carotid artery (ICA) origin
CT Findings
- +/- Ca++ in vessel wall
- Large plaques may show low density foci
MR Findings
- MRA provides multidirectional imaging (vs. conventional DSA)
- "Flow gap" (recovery of signal) in cases of high-grade stenosis
- Signal loss can occur if artery narrowed (>95%) but not occluded
- Brain T2WI, FLAIR may show "rosary-like" lesions in centrum semiovale ipsilateral to stenosis (hemodynamic failure?)
Other Modality Findings
- CTA
  - Demonstrates lumen
  - Wall Ca++ identified
  - Patchy/homogeneous low density in wall often seen with large necrotic/lipid plaque
  - Poor correlation with ulceration
- DSA
  - Current standard of reference (N.B.: Enhanced CTA, MRA adequate for evaluation of carotid stenosis)
  - Role of DSA
    - Evaluate great vessel origins
    - Calculate % carotid stenosis

Carotid Stenosis

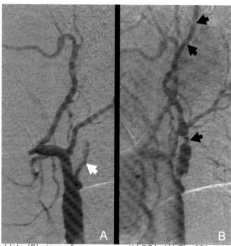

Early (A) and late (B) views of common carotid DSA. (A) The ICA appears occluded (white arrow). (B) Very slow filling of cervical ICA, the carotid "string sign," is present (B, arrows).

- At least 4 projections (AP, lat, both obliques) recommended
- Maximum narrowing used
  - Identify "tandem" distal ICA stenosis (2% of cases)
  - Depict presence of collateral flow (lower risk of stroke, TIA)
  - Detect other lesions (e.g., aneurysm)
- Calculating carotid stenosis
  - Methods vary (see "Atherosclerosis" for NASCET)
- Irregular plaque surface = increased stroke risk on medical Rx at all degrees of stenosis
- "Pseudoocclusion"
  - Very high-grade stenosis
  - Slow antegrade "trickle" of contrast may be shown only on late phase of angiogram
  - Important because endarterectomy an option if ICA still patent
  - High stroke risk

Imaging Recommendations
- U/S as screening tool
- CTA/MRA
- DSA if CTA/MRA show "occlusion"

Differential Diagnosis
Extrinsic Compressive Lesion (Rare)
- Carotid space neoplasm
Dissection
- Typically spares bulb, ICA origin (ASVD involves both)
- No Ca++

Pathology
General
- General Path Comments

o Significant ICA narrowing identified in 20%-30% of carotid territory strokes (vs. 5%-10% of general population)
- Etiology-Pathogenesis-Pathophysiology
  o Risk of stroke increases with stenosis severity
    ▪ Hypoperfusion?
    ▪ Artery-to-artery emboli
  o Stenosis is not sole factor (plaque morphology also correlated)

Gross Pathologic or Surgical Features
- See "Atherosclerosis"

Microscopic Features
- See "Atherosclerosis"

Clinical Issues

Presentation
- TIA
- Stroke (can be silent)

Natural History
- Progressive

Treatment & Prognosis
- NASCET
  o Symptomatic stenosis =/> 70% benefits from endarterectomy
  o Symptomatic moderate stenosis (50%-69%) also benefits from endarterectomy
- ACAS: Asymptomatic patients benefit even with stenosis of 60%

Selected References
1. Randoux B et al: Carotid artery stenosis: Prospective comparison of CT, Gadolinium-enhanced MR, and conventional angiography. Radiology 220: 179-85, 2001
2. Rothwell PM et al: Interrelation between plaque surface morphology and degree of stenosis on carotid angiograms and the risk of ischemic stroke in patients with symptomatic carotid stenosis. Stroke 31: 615-21, 2000
3. Rothwell PM et al: Critical appraisal of the design and reporting of studies of imaging and measurement of carotid stenosis. Stroke 31: 1444-50, 2000

Dissection

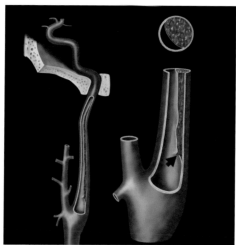

Graphic depicts subintimal dissection of the cervical ICA. Note proximal intimal tear (arrow), eccentric ICA narrowing. The bulb is spared and the dissection ends at the skull base.

Key Facts
- ICA = most frequent site of head/neck dissection
- Dissection causes 10%-25% of ischemic strokes in young adults
- Consider in young/middle-aged patient with headache, TIA

Imaging Findings
General Features
- Best diagnostic sign= tubular narrowing that spares bulb, stops at skull base
- Secondary emboli, stroke common
CT Findings
- NECT
  - May be negative
  - +/- Hyperdense carotid space mass (dissecting aneurysm)
- CECT may show true, false lumen separated by linear lucency
MR Findings
- Crescentic intramural hematoma
  - Acute clot iso-, subacute hyperintense on T1-, T2WI
- Eccentrically narrowed residual lumen
  - May have absent/diminished "flow void"
  - Slow flow may cause intravascular signal
Other Modality Findings
- Angiography (DSA/CTA/MRA)
  - ICA dissection usually spares bulb, ends at skull base
  - Smooth/irregular tapered narrowing +/- intimal flap
  - May have extralumenal pouch (dissecting aneurysm)
  - May occlude true lumen
Imaging Recommendations
- MR (fat-suppressed T1WI helpful for subacute clot), MRA
- DSA if MR/MRA negative

Dissection

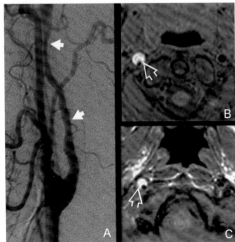

(A) DSA of a typical extracranial carotid dissection (arrows). Note sparing of bulb. (B, C) Axial fat-suppressed T1WI nicely demonstrates the high signal subacute hematoma in the carotid wall (open arrows).

Differential Diagnosis

Fibromuscular Dysplasia
- "String of beads" appearance > long tubular narrowing

Thrombosis
- Often involves bulb
- IA contrast may delineate intralumenal clot, meniscus

Atherosclerosis
- Involves bulb
- Irregular > smooth tapered narrowing
- Ca++ often present

Vasospasm (Migraine, Catheter-Induced, etc.)

Pathology

General
- General Path Comments
  - Can occur between or within any layers
    - Subintimal > subadventitial
  - Mid-cervical ICA > VA (skull base/C1, C1-2 most common)
    - 15% multiple vessels
  - Rare: Intracranial dissection
- Etiology-Pathogenesis
  - Congenital/acquired defect in internal elastic lamina
  - Trauma
    - Penetrating or blunt, stretching/torsion (including chiropractic manipulation which affects VA > ICA)
    - Minor neck torsion, trivial trauma in 25% (intense physical activity, coughing, sneezing)
  - "Spontaneous"
    - Underlying vasculopathy common (e.g., FMD, Marfan, Ehlers-Danlos)

- Familial ICA dissection may occur
- Hypertension in 1/3 of all patients
- Epidemiology
  - Annual incidence = 3.5 per 100,000

Gross Pathologic or Surgical Features
- Long segment narrowing with intramural clot

Clinical Issues

Presentation
- 70% of patients between 35-50y
- M = F
- Headache, neck/facial pain
  - 60%-90% of patients with cervical ICA dissection
  - Onset a few hours up to 3-4 weeks
- Horner's in 1/3
- Uncommon: Cranial nerve palsy (CN XII>IX, X, XI)
- Ischemic symptoms may occur as complication

Natural History
- Usually resolves spontaneously (6-8 weeks)

Treatment & Prognosis
- Treatment: Antithrombotics
- Prognosis
  - No residual or mild neurologic deficit in 70%
  - Disabling in 25%
  - Fatal in 5%

Selected References
1. Iu PP, Lam HS: Migrainous spasm simulating carotid dissection: A pitfall in MR arteriographic findings. AJNR 22: 1550-2, 2001
2. Lee WW et al: Bilateral internal carotid artery dissection due to trivial trauma. J Emerg Med 19: 35-41, 2000
3. Oelerich M et al: Craniocervical artery dissection: MR imaging and MR angiographic findings. Eur Radiol 9: 1385-91, 1999

NEOPLASMS

Low Grade Astrocytoma

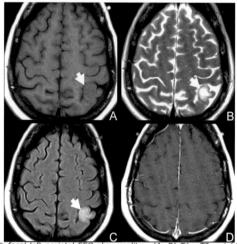

Patient with focal left parietal EEG abnormality. (A, B) T1-, T2-weighted and (C) FLAIR scans show small mass in the subcortical WM (arrows). (D) No enhancement is seen. Grade II fibrillary astrocytoma.

Key Facts
- Well-differentiated but infiltrating neoplasm, slow growth pattern
- May appear circumscribed on imaging but isn't (tumor cells often found beyond imaged signal abnormality)
- Intrinsic tendency for malignant progression, degeneration into anaplastic astrocytoma (AA)

Imaging Findings
General Features
- Homogeneous mass with some enlargement/distortion of affected structures
- Best diagnostic sign = focal/diffuse nonenhancing WM mass

CT Findings
- NECT
  - Ill-defined homogeneous hypo-/isodense mass
  - 20% Ca++
  - Cysts rare
- CECT: None (enhancement should raise suspicion of focal malignant degeneration)

MR Findings
- Signal intensity
  - Most common: Homogeneously hypointense T1WI; hyperintense T2WI/FLAIR
  - Less common: Ca++, cyst
  - Rare: Hemorrhage, surrounding edema
- May expand adjacent cortex
- May appear circumscribed but infiltrates adjacent brain
- Usually no enhancement; enhancement suggests progression to higher grade

Low Grade Astrocytoma

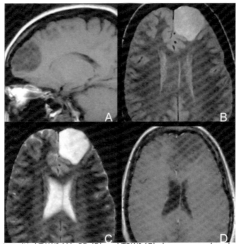

Pre-contrast sagittal T1WI (A), PD (B) and T2WI (C) show a very sharply demarcated frontal cortical/subcortical mass that doesn't enhance (D). Surgery disclosed unresectable grade II astrocytoma with tumor extending far beyond the imaged abnormalities.

Other Modality Findings
- DWI: Restricted diffusion usually absent
- MRS
  - High choline, low NAA
  - High MI/Cr ratio (0.82 +/- 0.25)
  - May delineate tumor extent better than conventional MR
- Dynamic contrast-enhanced T2*-weighted imaging: Relatively lower rCBV compared to AA, GBM

Differential Diagnosis
Anaplastic Astrocytoma
- Hemispheric WM lesion, usually non-enhancing
- May be indistinguishable without biopsy
Ischemia
- Vascular territory, + diffusion restriction (acute/early subacute)
Cerebritis
- Edema, patchy enhancement characteristic
- Usually shows restricted diffusion

Pathology
General
- General Path Comments
  - Location
    - Supratentorial 2/3 (frontal 1/3, temporal lobes 1/3)
    - Infratentorial 1/3 (brainstem; 50% of brainstem "gliomas" are low-grade astrocytoma)
- Genetics
  - TP53 mutation >60%
  - Overexpression of PDGFR-alpha

Low Grade Astrocytoma

- o Chromosomal abnormalities: Gain of 7q; 8q amplification; LOH 10p, 22q; chromosome 6 deletions
- Etiology-Pathogenesis-Pathophysiology
  - o Arise from differentiated astrocytes or astrocytic precursor cells
- Epidemiology
  - o Represents 25-30% of gliomas in adults
  - o 10-15% of all astrocytomas
  - o 2nd most common astrocytoma of childhood (pilocytic is 1st)

Gross Pathologic, Surgical Features
- Enlargement, distortion of invaded structures
- Infiltrating mass with blurring of GM/WM interface
- May appear grossly circumscribed but diffusely infiltrates adjacent brain
- Occasional cysts, Ca++

Microscopic Features
- Well differentiated fibrillary or gemistocytic neoplastic astrocytes
- Background of loosely structured, often microcystic tumor matrix
- Moderately increased cellularity
- Occasional nuclear atypia
- Mitotic activity generally absent or very rare
- **No** microvascular proliferation or necrosis
- Histologic variants
  - o Fibrillary
  - o Gemistocytic
  - o Protoplasmic
- MIB-1 low (< 4%)
- GFAP +

Staging or Grading Criteria
- WHO grade II

Clinical Issues

Presentation
- Peak incidence 30-40 yrs, mean age: 34 yrs
- M=F
- Seizures, increased ICP common presenting symptoms

Natural History
- Patients rarely succumb to spread of low grade tumor
- Inherent tendency for malignant progression to AA
- Recurrent disease associated with dedifferentiation in 50-75% cases

Treatment & Prognosis
- Median survival 6-10 yrs
- Treatment: Resection, +/- chemotherapy, XRT
- Increased survival: Young age, gross total resection
- Prognosis worse for pontine, better for medullary (especially dorsally exophytic) tumors

Selected References
1. Castillo M et al: Correlation of Myo-inositol levels and grading of cerebral astrocytomas. AJNR 21:1645, 2000
2. Kleihues P et al: Diffuse Astrocytoma. In Kleihues P, Cavenee WK (eds), Tumours of the Central Nervous System, 22-6. IARC Press, 2000
3. Knopp EA et al: Glial neoplasms: Dynamic contrast-enhanced T2*-weighted MR imaging. Radiology 211:791-8, 1999

Anaplastic Astrocytoma (AA)

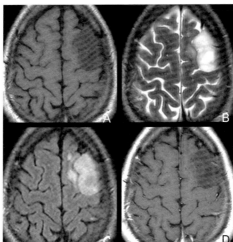

Pre- (A) and post-contrast (D) T1WI as well as T2WI (B) and FLAIR scans (C) show a rather well-delineated left posterior frontal mass that involves both the cortex and subcortical WM. Anaplastic astrocytoma (WHO grade III).

Key Facts
- Diffusely infiltrating hemispheric mass, variable imaging features
- Intermediate between diffuse astrocytoma (WHO grade II), GBM (IV)
- Neoplastic cells almost always found beyond areas of abnormal signal intensity

Imaging Findings
General Features
- Ill defined hemispheric WM mass
- Best diagnostic sign = nonenhancing infiltrating mass that predominately involves WM

CT Findings
- NECT
  - Low density mass
  - Ca++ rare
- CECT: Most don't enhance

MR Findings
- Variable signal intensity
  - Mixed iso- to hypointense on T1WI
  - Heterogeneously hyperintense T2WI/ FLAIR
  - Rare: Ca++, blood products, cysts
- Enhancement
  - Usually none; focal, nodular, homogeneous, patchy reported
  - Any enhancement should be suspicious for GBM!

Other Modality Findings
- MRS: Elevated Cho/Cr ratio, decreased NAA
- Dynamic contrast-enhanced T2*-weighted imaging: Elevated maximum rCBV compared to low grade astrocytoma

Imaging Recommendations
- MR (including contrast) + MRS

Anaplastic Astrocytoma (AA)

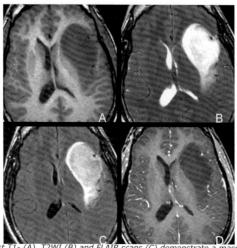

Pre-contrast T1- (A), T2WI (B) and FLAIR scans (C) demonstrate a mass infiltrating the left insula. (D) Post-contrast T1WI shows no enhancement. Anaplastic astrocytoma (WHO grade III).

Differential Diagnosis

Lower Grade Glioma
- Discrete
- May be indistinguishable without biopsy

Glioblastoma Multiforme (GBM)
- 95% necrotic core, enhancing rim

Cerebritis
- Patchy enhancement
- +/- Diffusion restriction

Ischemia
- Vascular territory
- Restricted diffusion if acute/subacute

Pathology

General
- General Path Comments
  - Location: Hemispheric WM, frontal & temporal lobes common
- Genetics
  - High frequency of TP53 mutations (>70%)
  - Abnormal cell cycle regulatory genes
  - p16 deletion, RB alterations, p19ARF deletion, CDK4 amplification
  - PTEN/MMAC1 mutations
  - Loss of heterozygosity: Chromosome 10q, 19q, 22q
  - Deletion of chromosome 6 (30%)
- Etiology-Pathogenesis-Pathophysiology
  - Usually evolves from diffuse astrocytoma (WHO II)
  - Occasionally arises **de novo**
- Epidemiology
  - 25% of gliomas
  - 1/3 of astrocytomas

Anaplastic Astrocytoma (AA)

Gross Pathologic, Surgical Features
- Infiltrating mass with poorly delineated margins
- Often expands invaded structures
- May appear discrete but tumor **always** infiltrates adjacent brain
- Cysts, hemorrhage uncommon

Microscopic Features
- Increased cellularity
- Marked mitotic activity
- Distinct nuclear atypia
- High nuclear/cytoplasmic ratio
- Nuclear/cytoplasmic pleomorphism
- Coarse nuclear chromatin
- **No** necrosis or microvascular proliferation
- GFAP + common
- MIB-1: 5-10%
- Gemistocytic variant can occur

Staging or Grading Criteria
- WHO grade III

Clinical Issues

Presentation
- Mean age 40-50y
- M:F = 1.8:1
- Varies with location
  - ○ Seizures, focal neurologic deficit common
  - ○ May have headache, other symptoms of raised ICP

Natural History
- Progression to secondary GBM common
- Commonly arises as recurrence after resection of a grade II tumor
- Spreads along white matter tracts
- Other sites: Ependyma, leptomeninges, CSF

Treatment & Prognosis
- Median survival 2–3 years
- Treatment: Resection and XRT, +/- chemotherapy
- Increased survival: Younger age, high Karnofsky score, gross total resection

Selected References
1. Wild-Bode C et al: Molicular determinants of glioma cell migration and invasion. J Neurosurg 94: 978-84, 2001
2. Kleihues P et al: Anaplastic Astrocytoma. In Kleihues P, Cavenee WK (eds), Tumours of the Central Nervous System, 27-8. IARC Press, 2000.
3. Rutherfood GS et al: Contrast enhanced imaging is critical to glioma nosology and grading. IJNR 1: 28-38, 1995

Glioblastoma Multiforme (GBM)

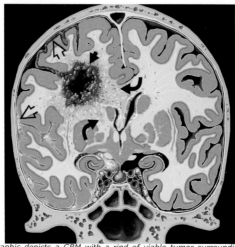

Coronal graphic depicts a GBM with a rind of viable tumor surrounding a central necrotic core (black arrow). Spread of tumor via compact WM tracts (curved arrows), subarachnoid and subpial spaces (open arrows), and ependyma is illustrated.

Key Facts
- Most common primary brain tumor
- Two types, primary (de novo) and secondary (degeneration from lower grade astrocytoma) GBM

Imaging Findings
General Features
- Poorly-marginated, diffusely-infiltrating hemispheric mass
- Best diagnostic sign = thick, irregular-enhancing rind of neoplastic tissue surrounding necrotic core (seen in 95%)

CT Findings
- NECT: Rim iso-, center hypodense; +/- hemorrhage; Ca++ rare
- CECT: Strong but inhomogeneous, irregular enhancement

MR Findings
- Variable signal (often mixed)
  - Iso-, hypointense on T1WI (may have subacute hemorrhage)
  - Hyperintense with adjacent vasogenic edema on T2WI, FLAIR
    - Viable tumor extends **far** beyond signal abnormalities!
  - Susceptibility artifact on T2* common
- Dynamic macromolecular, contrast-enhanced MR depicts microvascular permeability, may help assess tumor grade

Other Modality Findings
- DSA: Hypervascular with prominent tumor blush, A-V shunting
- MRS: Decreased NAA, MI; elevated Cho/Cr, lactate/water ratios
- DWI: Lower **measured** ADC than low-grade gliomas
- PWI: Distinguish GBM, low grade tumors (GBM has high rCBV)
- ^{201}Tl, ^{123}I-IMT show high uptake

Imaging Recommendations
- MR (include contrast-enhanced), MRS

Glioblastoma Multiforme (GBM)

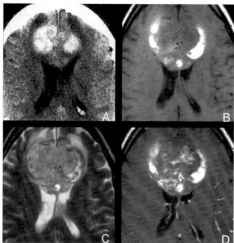

(A) NECT scan shows a hemorrhagic mass in both medial frontal lobes. Pre- (B) and post-contrast (D) T1WI as well as T2WI (C) show the extensive mass has patchy enhancement. "Butterfly" glioblastoma multiforme (WHO grade IV).

Differential Diagnosis
Other Neoplasm
- Anaplastic astrocytoma (usually doesn't enhance; enhancing foci may indicate degeneration into grade IV tumor)
- Metastasis

Non-neoplastic Ring-enhancing Mass
- Abscess (MRS shows metabolites such as succinate, amino acids)
- "Tumefactive" demyelination ("horseshoe"-shaped, incomplete enhancing ring, open towards cortex)

Pathology
General
- General Path Comments
  - Two genetically distinct GBM types, same appearance
  - Reddish-gray "rind" of tumor surrounds necrotic core
- Genetics
  - Primary GBM
    - Older patients, biologically more aggressive
    - Develops **de novo** (without pre-existing lower grade tumor)
    - Amplification, overexpression of EGFR, MDM2
    - PTEN mutation
    - Chromosome 10p loss of heterozygosity (LOH)
  - Secondary GBM
    - Younger patients, less aggressive than 1° GBM
    - Develops from lower grade astrocytoma
    - TP53 mutations
    - PDGFR amplification, overexpression
    - Chromosomes 10q, 17p LOH
    - Increased telomerase activity and hTERT expression

Glioblastoma Multiforme (GBM)

- Etiology-Pathogenesis-Pathophysiology
  - Occurs sporadically or as part of heritable tumor syndrome
    - NF-1
    - Turcot, Li-Fraumeni syndromes
  - Spreads by creating "permissive environment"
    - Produces proteases
    - Deposits extracellular matrix (ECM) molecules
    - Expresses integrins (neoangiogenesis, cellular invasion)
    - Neoplastic cells adhere to ECM, detach, migrate, proliferate
- Epidemiology
  - Most common primary brain tumor
  - 12%-15% of all intracranial neoplasms
  - 50%-60% of astrocytomas
  - Multifocal in up to 20% (2%-5% synchronous independent tumors)

Gross Pathologic or Surgical Features
- Most GBMs have marked vascularity
- +/- Gross hemorrhage

Microscopic Features
- Necrosis, microvascular proliferation = histologic hallmarks
- Pleomorphic astrocytes
- Marked nuclear atypia
- Numerous mitoses
- "Gemistocytic" astrocytes = large eosinophilic cells, spherical nuclei
- Low GFAP expression, high MIB-1

Staging or Grading Criteria
- WHO grade IV

Clinical Issues

Presentation
- Varies with location (seizure common)
- Peak 45-70y but may occur at any age

Natural History
- Relentless progression
- Patterns of dissemination
  - Most common = along white matter tracts, perivascular spaces
  - Less common = ependymal/subpial spread, CSF metastases
  - Uncommon: Dural/skull invasion
  - Rare: Extraneural spread (lung, liver, lymph nodes, bone)

Treatment & Prognosis
- Biopsy/tumor debulking followed by XRT
- Prognosis dismal (death in 9-12 months)
- Independent predictors of longer survival
  - Age (younger)
  - Karnofsky Performance Scale (higher)
  - Extent of resection (gross total vs. subtotal)
  - Degree of necrosis, enhancement on pre-operative MR

Selected References
1. Lacroix M et al: A multivariate analysis of 416 patients with GBM: Prognosis, extent of resection, and survival. J Neurosurg 95: 190-8, 2001
2. Ludemann L et al: Comparison of dynamic contrast-enhanced MRI with WHO tumor grading for gliomas. Eur Radiol 11: 1231-41, 2001
3. Kleihues P et al: Genetics of glioma progression and the definition of primary and secondary glioblastoma. Brain Pathol 7: 1131-6, 1997

Gliomatosis Cerebri (GC)

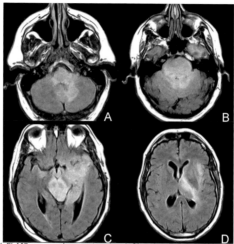

(A-D) Axial FLAIR scans show extensive infiltrating mass in the medulla, pons, midbrain, left temporal lobe and thalamus. Gliomatosis cerebri.

Key Facts
- Rare but important diffusely infiltrating glial tumor that can be mistaken for white matter microvascular disease
- GC involves two or more lobes

Imaging Findings
General Features
- Infiltrates, enlarges yet preserves underlying brain architecture
- Two or more lobes, diffuse white matter plus
  - Basal ganglia, thalami (75%)
  - Corpus callosum (50%)
  - Brainstem, spinal cord (10%-15%)
  - Cerebellum (10%)

CT Findings
- NECT: Poorly defined, asymmetric, low density (may be subtle)
- CECT: Usually doesn't enhance

MR Findings
- MR >> CT
- Iso-/hypodense on T1WI
- Hyperintense on T2WI, FLAIR
- Minimal enhancement; focus may represent malignant glioma

Other Modality Findings
- MRS: Elevated Cho/Cr, Cho/NAA; +/- lactate, lipid peaks
- FDG PET: Marked hypometabolism

Imaging Recommendations
- MR, MRS

Differential Diagnosis
White Matter Disease (Aging Brain, Microvascular Disease)
- No mass effect
- Some cases may be indistinguishable without biopsy!

Gliomatosis Cerebri (GC)

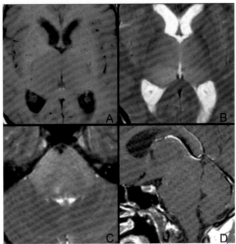

Axial pre-contrast T1- (A) and T2WI (B,C) show a bithalamic mass and pontine mass with mild obstructive hydrocephalus. (D) Sagittal post-contrast T1WI shows no enhancement. Gliomatosis cerebri caused by grade II fibrillary astrocytoma.

Astrocytoma, Other Glial Tumor
- GBM usually enhances; GC often doesn't
- May be indistinguishable without biopsy

Infection, Inflammation
- More acute presentation
- +/- Meningeal involvement

Pathology

General
- General Path Comments
  - Diffuse neoplastic overgrowth
  - Underlying brain architecture preserved
  - Two or more lobes
- Genetics
  - Karyotype consistent with clonal neoplasm arising from single cell
    - Chromosomal changes different from astrocytoma
    - May belong to separate category of brain tumor
- Etiology-Pathogenesis
  - Controversial (classified as neoplasm of unknown histogenesis)
  - Shares some, but not all, features of diffusely infiltrating astrocytoma
- Epidemiology
  - Rare
  - Peak incidence between 40-50y

Gross Pathologic or Surgical Features
- Two gross GC types recognized
  - Type I: Neoplastic overgrowth/ expansion of existing structures without circumscribed tumor mass
  - Type II: Diffuse lesion + focal neoplastic mass

Gliomatosis Cerebri (GC)

<u>Microscopic Features</u>
- Neuroepithelial neoplasm
- Elongated glial cells with hyperchromatic nuclei, variable mitoses
- Neoplastic cells often arranged in parallel rows
- Diffuse infiltration along, between myelinated nerve fibers
- Microvascular proliferation, necrosis usually absent
- Often GFAP+
- Ki-67 labelling index correlates with survival time
- Predominant cell type occasionally oligodendroglioma

<u>Staging or Grading Criteria</u>
- Usually WHO grade III

Clinical Issues
<u>Presentation</u>
- Nonspecific progressive neurological symptoms
  - Corticospinal tract deficits
  - Dementia, personality changes
  - Headache, seizures
  - Cranial neuropathy

<u>Natural History</u>
- Relentless progression

<u>Treatment & Prognosis</u>
- Stereotaxic biopsy (enhancing nodule, if present)
- Poor response to chemotherapy, XRT
- Poor prognosis
  - 50% mortality at 1 year
  - 75% by 3 years

Selected References
1. Rust P et al: Gliomatosis cerebri: Pitfalls in diagnosis. J Clin Neurosci 8: 361-3, 2001
2. Bendszus M et al: MR spectroscopy in gliomatosis cerebri. AJNR 21: 375-80, 2000
3. Lantos PL et al: Gliomatosis cerebri. In Kleihues P, Cavanee WK (eds), Tumours of the Central Nervous System, 92-3, IARC Press, 2000

Pilocytic Astrocytoma (PA)

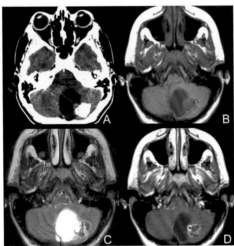

(A)CECT scan shows a cystic posterior fossa mass with enhancing nodule. Pre-contrast T1- (B) and T2-weighted MR scans show the cyst is hyperintense compared to CSF. (D) Post-contrast T1WI shows inhomogeneous enhancement of the nodule.

Key Facts
- Most common brain tumor in children
- Circumscribed, slowly growing
- Cerebellum > adjacent to 3rd ventricle > brainstem

Imaging Findings
General Features
- Best diagnostic signs
  - Cystic cerebellar mass with mural nodule
  - Enlarged optic nerve/chiasm/tract

CT Findings
- NECT
  - Discrete cystic/solid vermian or hemispheric mass
  - No surrounding edema
  - Hypo- to isodense
  - Ca++ 20%
  - Hemorrhage rare
  - May cause obstructive hydrocephalus
- CECT
  - > 95% enhance (patterns vary)
    - 50% nonenhancing cyst, strongly enhancing mural nodule
    - 40% solid with necrotic center, heterogeneous enhancement
    - 10% solid, homogeneous

MR Findings
- Solid/nodular portion usually hypo- to isointense T1WI; hyperintense T2WI
- Cyst hyperintense to CSF on T1WI, PD; doesn't suppress with FLAIR
- Intense but heterogeneous enhancement
- Leptomeningeal spread, enhancement can occur

Pilocytic Astrocytoma (PA)

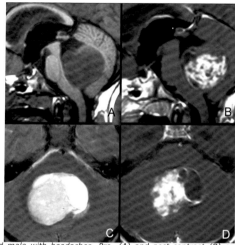

10-year-old male with headaches. Pre- (A) and post-contrast (B) sagittal T1WI, axial T2- (C) and post-contrast T1WI show a midline posterior fossa mass that is partially solid, partially cystic, with variegated contrast enhancement. Pilocytic astrocytoma.

<u>Other Modality Findings</u>
- MRS: High choline, low NAA, high lactate; high MI/Cr

Differential Diagnosis
<u>Medulloblastoma (PNET-MB)</u>
- Hyperdense, solid, midline mass fills fourth ventricle
- Heterogeneous enhancement
<u>Ependymoma</u>
- "Plastic" tumor, extends out 4th ventricle foramina
- Ca++, cysts, hemorrhage common; heterogeneous enhancement
<u>Ganglioglioma</u>
- Discrete, solid/cystic, cortically-based enhancing mass
- Ca++ common
<u>Pleomorphic Xanthoastrocytoma (PXA)</u>
- Enhancing nodule abuts pial surface
- Temporal lobe most common site
<u>Hemangioblastoma</u>
- Wrong age!
<u>Demyelination</u>
- Acute MS, ADEM can mimic optic nerve glioma

Pathology
<u>General</u>
- General Path Comments
  - Location
    - Common: Cerebellum (60%), optic nerve/optic chiasm/ hypothalamus (25-30%)
    - Less common: Brainstem, thalamus, basal ganglia
    - Uncommon: Cerebral hemisphere
  - May seed subarachnoid space

Pilocytic Astrocytoma (PA)

- Genetics
  - Syndromic: Association with NF-1
    - 15% of NF-1 patients develop PAs
    - Up to 1/3 of patients with optic pathway PAs have NF-1
  - Sporadic: No definite loss of tumor suppressor gene identified
- Etiology-Pathogenesis-Pathophysiology
  - Astrocytic precursor cell
- Epidemiology
  - > 80% under 20y
  - Most common astrocytoma in children
  - 5-10% of gliomas

Gross Pathologic, Surgical Features
- Well-circumscribed, soft, gray mass +/- cyst

Microscopic Features
- Classic "biphasic" pattern
  - Compacted bipolar cells with Rosenthal fibers
  - Loose-textured multipolar cells with microcysts, eosinophilic granular bodies
- Highly vascular with glomeruloid features
- Leptomeningeal seeding can occur
- MIB-1 = 0 – 3.9% (mean 1.1%)

Staging or Grading Criteria
- WHO grade I

Clinical Issues

Presentation
- Peak incidence: 1st – 2nd decades
- M=F
- H/A, N&V (increased ICP), visual loss (optic pathway lesions)

Natural History
- Slowly growing; may stabilize or even regress/involute
- Rare: Tumor may spread, still WHO grade I

Treatment & Prognosis
- Median survival rates at 20y = 70%
- Treatment
  - Cerebellar: Resection; +/- chemotherapy, +/- XRT
  - Opticochiasmatic/hypothalamic: Often none

Selected References
1. Burger PC et al: Pilocytic astrocytoma. In Kleihues P, Cavenee WK (eds), Tumours of the Central Nervous System, 45-51. IARC Press, 2000
2. Castillo M et al: Correlation of Myo-inositol levels and grading of cerebral astrocytomas. AJNR 21:1645-9, 2000
3. Hwang JH et al: Proton MR spectroscopic characteristics of pediatric pilocytic astrocytomas. AJNR 19:535-540, 1998

Pleomorphic Xanthoastrocytoma

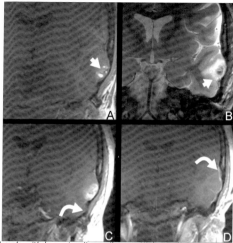

18-year-old male with long-standing epilepsy. High-resolution pre-contrast coronal T1- (A), T2WI (B) show a calcified cortical mass (arrows). Note adjacent skull remodeling. (C, D) The mass, adjacent meninges (curved arrows) enhance. PXA (WHO grade II).

Key Facts
- Distinct type of (usually) benign supratentorial astrocytoma found almost exclusively in young adults
- Cystic mass with mural nodule abutting meninges
- Rare but important cause of temporal lobe epilepsy

Imaging Findings
General Features
- Peripherally located hemispheric mass
  - 50%-60% cyst + mural nodule that abuts meninges
- Minimal/no perifocal edema
- Best diagnostic sign= supratentorial intracortical mass + adjacent "dural tail"

CT Findings
- NECT
  - Cystic = hypodense with mixed density nodule
  - Solid = variable (can be hypo-, hyperdense or mixed)
  - Ca++, hemorrhage, skull erosion rare
- CECT: Strong sometimes heterogeneous enhancement

MR Findings
- Low or mixed signal intensity on T1WI
- High or mixed signal intensity on T2WI, FLAIR
- Enhancement usually moderate/strong, well-delineated; +/- dural "tail"
- Some cases have associated cortical dysplasia

Other Modality Findings
- FDG-PET may show hypermetabolic foci even in low-grade PXAs

Imaging Recommendations
- MR + MRS

Pleomorphic Xanthoastrocytoma

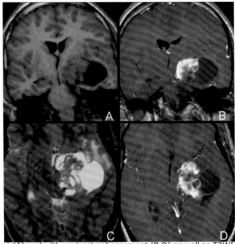

T1WI without (A) and with contrast enhancement (B,D) as well as T2WI (C) show an inhomogeneous partially enhancing temporal lobe mass. PXA (W.H.O. grade III).

Differential Diagnosis
Ganglioglioma
- Mural nodule often not adjacent to meninges

Pilocytic Astrocytoma
- Supratentorial location other than hypothalamus/chiasm rare
- No dural tail

Meningioma
- Usually older patients
- Meningioma-like lesion in young patient should raise suspicion of PXA

Other
- DNET
- Glioneuronal hamartoma

Pathology
General
- General Path Comments
  - Superficial location (often involves cortex, meninges)
  - 98% supratentorial
- Genetics
  - No definite association with hereditary tumor syndromes
  - Some PXAs with TP53 mutations reported
- Etiology-Pathogenesis
  - May originate from cortical (subpial) astrocytes
  - May arise from multipotential neuroectodermal precursor cells common to both neurons, astrocytes
- Epidemiology
  - <1% of all astrocytomas

Gross Pathologic or Surgical Features
- Cystic cortical mass with mural nodule abutting meninges

Microscopic Features
- Tumor sharply delineated from cortex

Pleomorphic Xanthoastrocytoma

- GFAP +
- Some PXAs are positive for synaptophysin, neurofilament proteins
- "Pleomorphic" appearance
  - Fibrillary and giant multinucleated neoplastic astrocytes
  - Large xanthomatous (lipid-containing) cells
  - Dense reticulin network
  - Lymphocytic infiltrates
- Necrosis, mitotic figures rare/absent
  - MIB generally <1%
- May be associated with cortical dysplasia

Staging or Grading Criteria
- WHO grade II
- PXA with anaplastic features
  - Significant mitoses (5 or more per 10 HPF)
  - +/- Necrosis

Clinical Issues

Presentation
- Majority with long-standing epilepsy
- Tumor of children, young adults
  - 2/3 < 18y
  - Has been reported from 2-66y
- M = F

Natural History
- Usually circumscribed, slow growing
- Aggressive PXA with malignant progression, dissemination occasionally occurs

Treatment & Prognosis
- Surgical resection
- 75% recurrence-free 5 year survival

Selected References
1. Kepes JJ et al: Pleomorphic xanthoastrocytoma. In Kleihues P, Cavenee WK (eds), Tumours of the Nervous System, 52-4, IARC Press, 2000
2. Russo CP et al: Pleomorphic xanthoastrocytoma: Report of two cases and review of the literature. IJNR 2: 570-8, 1996
3. Lipper MH et al: Pleomorphic xanthoastrocytoma, a distinctive astroglial tumor: Neuroradiologic and pathologic features. AJNR 14: 1397-1404, 1993

Oligodendroglioma

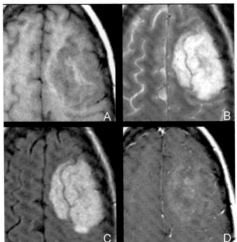

Pre-contrast T1- (A), T2WI (B), and FLAIR scans (C) show a well-delineated, cortically-based, posterior frontal mass. No surrounding edema is present. (D) Post-contrast T1WI shows minimal enhancement. Oligodendroglioma (WHO grade II).

Key Facts
- Well-differentiated, slowly growing but infiltrating tumor
- Typically involves cortex, subcortical white matter
- 20%-50% aggressive (anaplastic oligodendroglioma)

Imaging Findings
General Features
- Best diagnostic sign = partially Ca++ cortically-based mass in middle-aged adult
- May expand, erode calvarium

CT Findings
- NECT
  - Hypo-/isodense
  - Majority calcify
  - +/- Hemorrhage/cysts (20%)
- CECT: Enhancement varies from none to striking

MR Findings
- Often heterogeneous
  - Hypo-/isointense to GM on T1WI
  - Hyperintense on T2WI
  - Hemorrhage, necrosis rare unless anaplastic
- May appear well circumscribed with minimal associated edema
- 50% enhance

Differential Diagnosis
Astrocytoma
- Calcification less common
- Usually involve white matter, cortex relatively spared

Ganglioglioma
- Childhood, young adult tumor
- Usually temporal lobe, deep WM

132

Oligodendroglioma

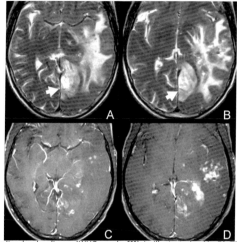

Anaplastic oligodendroglioma (WHO grade III) is illustrated. (A, B) T2WI show a cortically-based occipital mass (arrows) with extensive edema. (C, D) Post-contrast T1WIs show nodular enhancement, tumor spread.

- Sharply demarcated, commonly cystic
- Ca++ common

Dysembryoplastic Neuroepithelial Tumor (DNET)
- Childhood, young adult tumor
- Sharply demarcated cortical neoplasm
- Heterogeneous, "bubbly" appearance
- Heterotopic GM commonly associated

Pathology
General
- General Path Comments
  - Starts in cortex, grows into subcortical WM
  - Location: Majority supratentorial (85%)
    - Most common site = frontal lobe
    - May also involve temporal, parietal or occipital lobes
    - Posterior fossa rare
  - Well-differentiated and anaplastic types
  - Solid, infiltrative lesions
  - Variant = oligoastrocytoma (mixed tumor with 2 distinct neoplastic cell types)
- Genetics
  - Loss of heterozygosity for 1p and 19q (50-70%)
- Etiology-Pathogenesis
  - Arises from neoplastic transformation of mature oligodendrocytes or immature glial precursors
- Epidemiology
  - 5-10% of intracranial neoplasms
  - 5-25% of all gliomas

Gross Pathologic or Surgical Features
- Well-defined, grayish-pink soft mass
- Located in cortex, subcortical white matter

Oligodendroglioma

- Ca++ frequent
- +/- Cystic degeneration, hemorrhage
- Rare: Infiltrates leptomeninges

Microscopic Features
- Moderately cellular tumors with occasional mitoses
- Rounded, homogeneous nuclei and clear cytoplasm ("fried egg," honeycomb patterns probably artifactual)
- +/- Microcalcification, mucoid/cystic degeneration
- May have dense network of branching capillaries

Staging or Grading Criteria
- WHO grade II
- Anaplastic oligodendroglioma = WHO grade III
  o Numerous mitoses
  o Microvascular proliferation
  o Necrosis +/-

Clinical Issues

Presentation
- Peak incidence 4th and 5th decade
- Slight male preponderance
- Patients have relatively long-standing history of symptoms
  o Most common = seizure, headache

Natural History
- Good outcome
  o Younger age
  o Frontal location
  o Lack of enhancement
  o Complete resection
- Worse prognosis
  o Necrosis
  o Mitotic activity, nuclear atypia
  o Cellular pleomorphism
  o Microvascular proliferation
- Local recurrence common; malignant progression may occur

Treatment & Prognosis
- Surgical resection with adjuvant chemotherapy +/- XRT
- Median post-operative survival times range 3-6 years
- 5-year survival rate 50%

Selected References
1. Reifenberger G et al: Oligodendroglioma. Anaplastic Oligodendroglioma. In Kleihues P, Cavenee WK (eds), Pathology & Genetics of Tumours of the Central Nervous System, 56-69. IARC Press, 2000
2. Prayson RA et al: Clinicopathologic Study of Forty-Four Histologically Pure Supratentorial Oligodendrogliomas. Ann Diagn Pathol 4:218-27, 2000
3. Fortin D et al: Oligodendroglioma: An Appraisal of Recent Data Pertaining to Diagnosis and Treatment. Neurosurgery 45:1279-91, 1999

Ependymoma

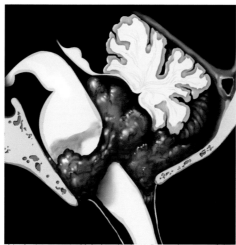

Sagittal graphic depicts a typical lobulated "plastic" ependymoma of the 4th ventricle. The tumor extrudes laterally through the foramina of Luschka into the CPAs and posteroinferiorly through Magendie into the cisterna magna.

Key Facts
- Slowly growing tumor of children, young adults
- Third most common childhood posterior fossa mass
- Arises from ependymal cells or ependymal rests

Imaging Findings
General Features
- Best diagnostic sign = "plastic" tumor squeezes out 4th ventricle foramina into CPAs, cisterna magna
CT Findings
- NECT
  - Infratentorial (children < 3y)
    - Floor of 4th ventricle, extends into CPA/cisterna magna
    - Majority isodense with brain
    - Ca++ common (50%); +/- cysts, hemorrhage
  - Supratentorial (children >3y, young adults)
    - Large heterogeneous parenchymal > peri-/intraventricular mass
    - Ca++ common (50%)
  - Hydrocephalus common
- CECT
  - Variable heterogeneous enhancement
MR Findings
- Heterogeneous
  - Slightly hypointense to brain on T1WI
  - Iso/hypointense on T2WI
  - Ca++, cysts, necrosis, blood products common
- Hydrocephalus (>90%)
- Moderate, heterogeneous enhancement
Other Modality Findings
- MRS: Higher NAA:Cho, Cr:Cho than astrocytomas, PNET-MB

Ependymoma

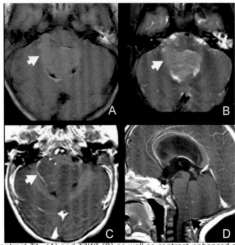

Axial pre-contrast T1- (A) and T2WI (B) as well as contrast-enhanced axial (C) and sagittal (D) MR scans show an ependymoma of the 4th ventricle extruding through the foramen of Lushka (arrows) into the right CPA cistern.

Differential Diagnosis

Medulloblastoma (PNET-MB)
- Hyperdense on NECT
- Homogeneous

Cerebellar Astrocytoma
- Cystic/solid
- Often off-midline

Brainstem Glioma
- Hypodense (often dorsally exophytic) brainstem mass
- Projects into, rather than originates from, 4th ventricle

Pathology

General
- General Path Comments
  - Location
    - 2/3rd infratentorial (floor of 4th ventricle)
    - 1/3rd supratentorial (parenchymal/periventricular > intraventricular)
  - 4 subtypes
    - Cellular
    - Papillary
    - Clear-cell
    - Tanycytic
  - May grow through ventricular wall, adhere to adjacent brain
- Genetics
  - Multiple described; most common = deletions, translocations of chromosome 22
  - NF-2 (multiple spinal ependymomas)
- Etiology-Pathogenesis
  - Possible link with SV40

Ependymoma

- Epidemiology
  - 8% - 15% of all intracranial tumors in children
  - Third most common posterior fossa tumor in children
  - Slight male predominance
  - Bimodal age distribution
    - Major peak = 1-5y
    - Second smaller peak = mid-30s

Gross Pathologic or Surgical Features
- Well demarcated
- Soft, lobulated, grayish-red mass
- +/- Cysts, necrosis, hemorrhage
- Extrudes through 4th ventricle outlet foramina
- Occasionally invades adjacent brain parenchyma

Microscopic Features
- Ependymoma
  - Perivascular pseudorosettes
  - True ependymal rosettes (less frequent)
  - Moderately cellular with low mitotic activity
  - Occasional nuclear atypia, occasional to no mitoses
  - S-100, vimentin +
- Anaplastic ependymoma
  - High cellularity
  - Nuclear atypia, hyperchromatism
  - Brisk mitotic activity
  - +/- Microvascular proliferation
  - Pseudopalisading with variable necrosis

Staging or Grading Criteria
- WHO grade II
- WHO grade III (anaplastic)

Clinical Issues

Presentation
- Common: Headache, nausea, vomiting
- Other
  - Ataxia, hemiparesis, visual disturbances, neck pain, torticollis, dizziness
  - Infants: Irritability, lethargy, developmental delay, vomiting, macrocephaly

Natural History
- 3%-17% CSF dissemination

Treatment & Prognosis
- Poor prognosis (5-year survival 50%-60%)
- Gross total resection correlates with improved survival
- Current treatment: Surgical resection +/- chemo, RT

Selected References
1. Smyth MD et al: Intracranial ependymomas of childhood: current management strategies. Pediatric Neurosurgery 33:138-50, 2000
2. Wiestler OD et al: Ependymoma. In Kleihues P, Cavanee WK (eds), Pathology & Genetics of Tumours of the Central Nervous System,72-7. IARC Press, 2000
3. Robertson PL et al: Survival and prognostic factors following radiation therapy and chemotherapy for ependymomas in children: a report of the Children's Cancer Group. J Neurosurg 88:695-703, 1998

Choroid Plexus Tumors

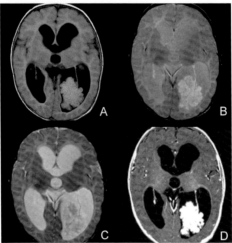

Axial FLAIR (A), PD- (B), T2WI (C) and contrast-enhanced SPGR (D) show a lobulated, intensely-enhancing mass in trigone (atrium) of the left lateral ventricle. The ventricles are markedly enlarged. Choroid plexus papilloma.

Key Facts
- Most frequent brain tumor in children <1y
- Two types, papilloma (CPP) and carcinoma (CPCa)
- Prevalence of CPP 4-8x CPCa
- Both CPPs and CPCa may spread via CSF

Imaging Findings
General Features
- Best diagnostic sign = child < 5y with lobulated, frond-like mass in trigone of lateral ventricle
- Hydrocephalus (obstructive or CSF over-production)

CT Findings
- NECT
  - 75% iso/hyperdense
  - Hydrocephalus
  - Punctate Ca++ in 25%
  - Occasional: Hemorrhage with blood-CSF level
  - Rare: Predominately cystic CPP
- CECT
  - Intense, homogeneous enhancement

MR Findings
- Mottled, iso/hypointense on T1WI
- Frond-like papillae with CSF in-between
- Intense enhancement
- Limited (focal) parenchymal invasion may occur with CPPs; extensive should raise suspicion of CPCa
- +/- "Flow voids," hemorrhage

Other Modality Findings
- U/S: Highly echogenic mass with irregular borders, hydrocephalus
- Color Doppler: May show vascular pedicle

Choroid Plexus Tumors

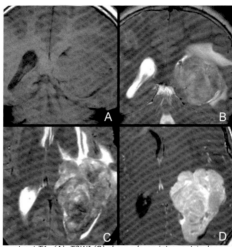

Coronal pre-contrast T1- (A), T2WI (B) show a large intraventricular mass. Axial T2-(C), post-contrast T1WI (D) show the inhomogeneous, strongly-enhancing mass invades the adjacent parenchyma. Choroid plexus carcinoma (courtesy G. Halvorsen).

- DSA
  - Enlarged choroidal arteries
  - Dense, prolonged vascular stain
  - A-V shunting common

Imaging Recommendations
- Contrast-enhanced MR of brain and spine prior to shunt, surgery

Differential Diagnosis
Villous Hypertrophy
- Diffuse enlargement of choroid in both lateral ventricles
- May be associated with hypersecretory hydrocephalus

Other Intraventricular Neoplasms/Cysts
- Metastasis, meningioma (rare in children unless NF-1)
- Ependymoma (ventricle uncommon supratentorial site)
- Xanthogranuloma (avascular, older patients)

Vascular Lesion
- AVM, cavernous angioma

Physiologic Enlargement
- Collateral venous drainage (e.g., Sturge-Weber)
- Post-surgical (temporal lobectomy)

Pathology
General
- General Path Comments
  - CPPs = cauliflower-like intraventricular mass
  - CPCas invade brain, may be necrotic
- Genetics
  - Li-Fraumeni, Aicardi syndromes (p53 mutations)
  - No known mutations in sporadic tumors

Choroid Plexus Tumors

- Etiology-Pathogenesis-Pathophysiology
  - SV40 virus-like DNA found in 50%
  - Hydrocephalus caused by CSF overproduction or obstruction (IVOH or EVOH secondary to hemorrhage, arachnoiditis)
- Epidemiology
  - 0.5% of all adult brain tumors
  - 2%-4% of all pediatric brain tumors
  - Most common brain tumor in children <1y

Gross Pathologic or Surgical Features
- Well-circumscribed frond-like/papillary intraventricular mass
- Cysts, hemorrhage common
- Atrium of lateral ventricle most common site in children; 4th ventricle and/or CPA in adults

Microscopic Features
- CPP
  - Fronds of cuboidal epithelial cells with fibrovascular core
  - No necrosis, hemorrhage, gross brain invasion
  - S-100 protein in 90%, GFAP + in 25%-50%
  - Immunohistochemistry: + Cytokeratins, vimentin
- CPCa
  - Increased cellularity (high nuclear:cytoplasm ratios)
  - Nuclear pleomorphism, frequent mitoses
  - Diffuse brain invasion common

Staging or Grading Criteria
- CPP = WHO grade I
- CPCa = WHO grade III

Clinical Issues

Presentation
- Signs of elevated ICP
- 75% < 10y (mean age = 5y)
- M > F

Natural History
- CPP = benign, slowly growing tumor
- CPCa = malignant
- **Both** CPP, CPCa may seed CSF

Treatment & Prognosis
- CPP = surgical resection
  - 5 year survival rate approaches 100%
- CPCa = resection + adjuvant chemotherapy
  - 5 yr survival rate = 25-40%

Selected References
1. Levy ML et al: Choroid plexus tumors in children: Significance of stromal invasion. Neurosurg 48: 303-9, 2001
2. Shin JH et al: Choroid plexus papilloma in the posterior cranial fossa: MR, CT, and angiographic findings. J Clin Imaging 25: 154-62, 2001
3. Aguzzi A et al: Choroid plexus tumors. In Kleihues P, Cavenee WK (eds): Tumours of the Nervous System, 84-6, IARC Press, 2000

Ganglioglioma

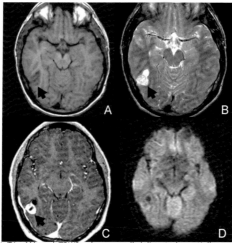

Pre-contrast T1- (A) and T2WIs show a well-delineated, partially cystic posterior temporal lobe mass (arrows). (C) Post-contrast thin section SPGR shows the nodule enhances. (D) DWI shows no restriction. Ganglioglioma.

Key Facts
- Mix of mature but neoplastic ganglion cells + neoplastic astrocytes
- Common neoplasm causing chronic temporal lobe epilepsy (TLE)
- Tumor of children, young adults

Imaging Findings
General Features
- Three patterns
  - Most common = circumscribed cyst + mural nodule
  - Solid tumor (often thickens, expands gyri)
  - Uncommon = infiltrating, poorly-delineated mass
- Best diagnostic sign= partially cystic, enhancing, cortically-based mass in child/young adult with TLE
CT Findings
- NECT
  - Variable density
    - 60% hypodense
    - 40% mixed hypo- (cyst), isodense (nodule)
    - 35-40 % Ca ++
  - Superficial lesions may expand, remodel bone
- CECT
  - Approximately 50% enhance
    - Varies from moderate, uniform to heterogeneous
    - Can be solid, rim or nodular
MR Findings
- Variable signal
  - Most are iso/hypointense relative to GM on T1WI
  - Mildly to moderately hyperintense on T2WI
- Doesn't suppress on FLAIR
- 50% enhance
  - Usually moderate but heterogeneous

Ganglioglioma

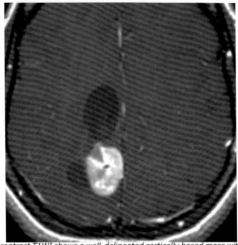

Axial post-contrast T1WI shows a well-delineated cortically based mass with enhancing nodule. Ganglioglioma was found at surgery.

- Associated cortical dysplasia in 50%

Other Modality Findings
- MRS: Elevated Cho/Cr
- FDG-PET: Usually decreased/normal but low grade GGs may have some hypermetabolic foci
- ^{201}Tl-SPECT: Increased activity in high grade

Imaging Recommendations
- MR, MRS

Differential Diagnosis
Other Neoplasm
- Pilocytic astrocytoma
- PXA
- Low grade fibrillary astrocytoma

Glioneuronal Hamartoma

Nonneoplastic Cyst
- Neurocysticercosis

Pathology
General
- General Path Comments
  - Most common mixed neuronal-glial tumor
  - Can occur anywhere
    - 80% temporal lobe, 10% frontal lobe
    - 10% other (brainstem, spinal cord)
  - Desmoplastic infantile ganglioglioma (DIG) may be very large, multicystic, with peripheral enhancing solid component
- Genetics
  - Sporadic
    - Tp53 mutations found in malignant degeneration
  - Syndromic: GG has been reported in Turcot syndrome

Ganglioglioma

- Etiology-Pathogenesis-Pathophysiology
  - Two theories
    - Neoplastic transformation of glial hamartoma or subpial granule cells
    - Differentiated remnants of embryonal neuroblastoma/PNETs
- Epidemiology
  - 1% of primary intracranial neoplasms
  - 80% of patients < 30y
  - M = F

Gross Pathologic or Surgical Features
- Solid or cystic mass with mural nodule
- Often expands cortex

Microscopic Features
- Dysmorphic, occasionally binucleate neurons
  - EM shows dense core granules, variable synapses
  - Immunohistochemistry
    - + For synaptophysin
    - Majority exhibit CD34 immunoreactivity
- Neoplastic glial cells (usually astrocytes)
  - GFAP +
  - Mitoses rare (75% have Ki-67 <1%, low MIB)

Staging or Grading Criteria
- WHO grade I or II
- Uncommon: Anaplastic ganglioglioma (WHO grade III)
- Rare: Malignant with GBM-like glial component (WHO IV)

Clinical Issues

Presentation
- > 90% chronic epilepsy

Natural History
- Well-differentiated tumor with slow growth pattern
- 5%-10% malignant degeneration (glial component)

Treatment & Prognosis
- Excellent prognosis if resection complete

Selected References
1. Hayashi Y et al: Malignant transformation of a gangliocytoma/ ganglioglioma into a glioblastoma multiforme: A molecular genetic analysis. J Neurosurg 95: 138-42, 2001
2. Nelson JS et al: Ganglioglioma and gangliocytoma. In Kleihues P, Cavenee WK, Tumours of the Nervous System, 96-98, IARC Press, 2000
3. Provenzale JM et al: Gangliogliomas: Characterization by registered PET-MR images. AJR 172: 1103-7, 1999

DNETs

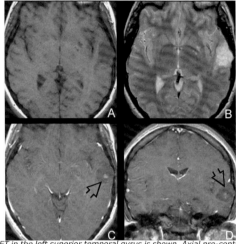

Classic DNET in the left superior temporal gyrus is shown. Axial pre-contrast T1- (A), T2WI (B) and post-contrast axial (C), coronal (D) T2WI show the "bubbly" lesion is sharply delineated, remodels the overlying calvarium. Faint enhancement is present (open arrows).

Key Facts
- Benign, focal intra cortical mass
- Often superimposed on background of cortical dysplasia
- Long-standing partial complex seizures in child/young adult typical

Imaging Findings
General Features
- Best diagnostic sign = "bubbly" cortical mass in young patient with long- standing seizures
- Minimal or no mass effect
- May remodel overlying bone
- Very slow growth over many years

CT Findings
- NECT
  - Wedge-shaped low density area
    - Cortical/subcortical
    - Extends towards ventricle (30%)
    - Scalloped inner table (60+%)
    - 20% Ca++
  - May resemble stroke (no temporal evolution to atrophy)
- CECT
  - 80% don't enhance
  - 20% faint nodular/patchy enhancement

MR Findings
- Pseudocystic, multinodular ("bubbly") mass
  - Well-circumscribed
  - Hypointense on T1WI
  - Thin, bright rim on PD
  - Very hyperintense on T2WI
  - Mixed (hypo/isointense) on FLAIR

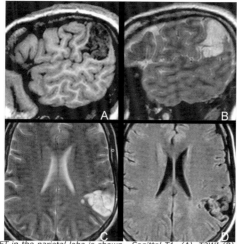

Classic DNET in the parietal lobe is shown. Sagittal T1- (A), T2WI (B), axial T2WI (C) and FLAIR scans (D) are illustrated.

- No peritumoral edema
- One-third show faint punctate/ring enhancement

Other Modality Findings
- 18F-FDG PET may demonstrate hypometabolism
- Ictal Tc99m-HMPAO SPECT may show hyperperfusion; interictal hypoperfusion
- MRS: Nonspecific

Differential Diagnosis

Ganglioma
- Ca++ common
- Strong enhancement

Pleomorphic Xanthoastrocytoma (PXA)
- Enhancing nodule abuts pia
- Look for dural "tail"

Pathology

General
- Genetics
  - Familial unknown, although focal cortical dysplasias may be syndrome-related
  - Reported cases with NF1
- Embryology
  - Probably originate from abnormal cells in germinal matrix
- Etiology-Pathogenesis-Pathophysiology
  - Dysplastic cells in germinal matrix
  - Extend along migratory path of neurons towards cortex
  - Associated cortical dysplasia common
- Epidemiology
  - Probably around 1%-2% of primary brain tumors in patients <20y
  - Reported in 5%-80% of epilepsy specimens

DNETs

Gross Pathologic or Surgical Features
- Thick gyrus
- Temporal lobe most common site
- Others: Parietal cortex, caudate

Microscopic Features
- Multinodular architecture
- Hallmark = "specific glioneuronal element"
  - Columns of heterogeneous cells oriented perpendicular to cortex
  - Oligodendrocyte-like cells arranged around capillaries
  - Other cells show astrocytic, neuronal differentiation
- Microcystic degeneration
  - Neurons "float" in pale, eosinophilic mucoid matrix
- Adjacent cortical dysplasia common
- Low proliferative potential with variable MIB-1 index

Staging or Grading Criteria
- WHO grade I

Clinical Issues

Presentation
- Partial complex seizures
- Children/young adults
- Typically identified before age 20

Natural History
- Benign lesions
- Don't progress/recur

Treatment & Prognosis
- Seizures may become intractable
- Surgical resection of epileptogenic foci (may include cortical dysplasia)

Selected References
1. Lee DY et al: Dysembryoplastic neuroepithelial tumor: Radiological findings (including PET, SPECT, and MRS) and surgical strategy. J Neurooncol 47: 167-74, 2000
2. Daumas-Duport C et al: Dysembryoplastic neuroepithelial tumors: In Kleihues P, Cavenee WK (eds), Tumors of the Nervous System, 103-6, IARC Press, 2000
3. Ostertun B et al: Dysembryoplastic neuroepithelial tumors: MR and CT evaluation. AJNR 17: 419-30, 1996

Central Neurocytoma

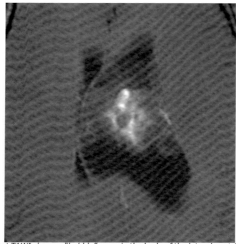

Post-contrast T1WI shows a "bubbly" mass in the body of the lateral ventricle attached to the septum pellucidum. Central neurocytoma.

Key Facts
- Neuroepithelial tumor with neuronal differentiation
- Intraventricular mass attached to septum pellucidum
- Characteristic "bubbly" appearance on imaging studies

Imaging Findings
General Features
- Best diagnostic sign= "bubbly" mass in frontal horn/body of lateral ventricle

CT Findings
- NECT
  - Usually mixed solid/cystic (iso-/hyperdense)
  - +/- Calcification (50%)
  - Hydrocephalus common
- CECT: Moderate, heterogeneous enhancement

MR Findings
- Heterogeneous; mostly isointense with cortex on T1WI
- Hyperintense, "bubbly" appearance on T2WI
- "Flow voids" in some cases
- Moderate to strong heterogeneous enhancement

Other Modality Findings
- MRS: Large Cho peak; unidentifiable peak at 3.55 ppm
- DSA: May be very vascular

Differential Diagnosis
Subependymoma
- Older patients
- Usually faint or no enhancement
- 4th > lateral ventricle

Ependymoma
- Supratentorial ependymomas rarely intraventricular

Central Neurocytoma

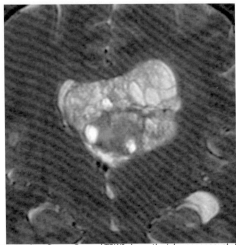

Same case as previous figure. Coronal T2WI shows the inhomogeneously hyperintense mass fills the lateral ventricle, does not invade adjacent brain. Central neurocytoma.

- Aggressive features

Giant Cell Astrocytoma
- May be indistinguishable from neurocytoma
- Look for stigmata of tuberous sclerosis
  - Subependymal nodules, cortical tubers, white matter lesions

Metastasis
- Uncommon, usually older patients
- Solid enhancement

Pathology
General
- General Path Comments
  - Location
    - >50% in frontal horn/body lateral ventricle
    - 15% extend into 3rd ventricle; 3% 3rd ventricle only
    - Both lateral ventricles 13%
    - Rare extraventricular tumors with neurocytoma features reported
  - Parenchymal invasion rare
- Etiology-Pathogenesis
  - May arise from neuronal or bipotential progenitor cells
- Epidemiology
  - <1% of all primary intracranial neoplasms
  - 10% of intraventricular neoplasms

Gross Pathologic or Surgical Features
- Grayish, friable, circumscribed, intraventricular mass
- Moderately vascular; may hemorrhage, calcify

Microscopic Features
- Resembles oligodendroglioma
- Uniform round cells with neuronal differentiation
  - Stippled nuclei, perinuclear halos

Central Neurocytoma

- Various architectural patterns (can resemble other neoplasms)
  - Monotonous sheets of cells
  - Perivascular pseudorosettes (ependymoma)
  - Honeycomb appearance (oligodendroglioma)
  - Large fibrillary areas (pineocytoma)
- Benign (low proliferation rate, mitoses rare)
- Anaplasia, necrosis rare
  - Occasionally have brisk mitotic activity
  - Microvascular proliferation
- Immunopositive for synaptophysin; rarely for GFAP

Staging or Grading Criteria
- WHO grade II

Clinical Issues

Presentation
- Young adults (20-40y)
- M=F
- Headache (hydrocephalus, increased ICP)
- Hydrocephalus secondary to foramen of Monro obstruction
- Tumors of septum, 3rd ventricle, hypothalamus may have visual disturbances, hormonal dysfunction

Natural History
- Usually benign
- Local recurrence may occur
- Craniospinal dissemination extremely rare

Treatment & Prognosis
- Complete surgical resection
- Gamma knife radiosurgery improves local control rates and increases survival
- 5-year survival rate = 80%

Selected References
1. Anderson RC et al: Radiosurgery for the treatment of recurrent central neurocytomas. Neurosuug 48: 1231-8, 2001
2. Figarella-Branger D et al: Central neurocytoma. In Kleihues P, Cavenee WK (eds), Pathology & Genetics of Tumours of the Nervous System, 107-9, IARC Press 2000
3. Kim DG et al: In vivo proton MRS of central neurocytoma. Neurosurg 46: 329-34, 2000

Meningioma

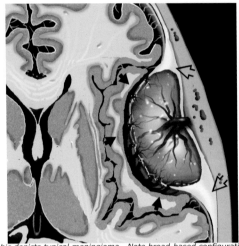

Axial graphic depicts typical meningioma. Note broad-based configuration, reactive bone with enostotic "spur," vascular pedicle, and CSF-vascular "cleft" (black arrows). Nonneoplastic dural thickening ("tail") is indicated by the open arrows.

Key Facts
- Most common nonglial primary brain tumor
- Most common intracranial extraaxial neoplasm in adults

Imaging Findings
General Features
- Extra-axial mass
  - Broad base towards dural surface
  - Cortex displaced (gray matter "buckled")
  - CSF-vascular "cleft"
- Best diagnostic sign= dual "tail" (but **not** pathognomonic!)

CT Findings
- NECT
  - Hyperostosis, irregular cortex, enostotic "spur" common
  - 70%-75% hyperdense
  - 20%-25% calcified
  - 2%-3% intra- or peritumoral cysts
- CECT: > 90% strong, uniform enhancement

MR Findings
- Usually isointense with cortex on all sequences
- 25% atypical (extensive necrosis, cysts, hemorrhage)
- Edema in 50%-65%
- > 95% strong enhancement; often heterogeneous
- Dural "tail"
  - 35%-80% of cases
  - Thickened dura tapers away from tumor

Other Modality Findings
- DWI, ADC maps: Appearance variable
- MRS: Cho/Cr ratio on MRS correlates with proliferative potential; Ala peak at 1.5ppm suggests meningioma

Meningioma

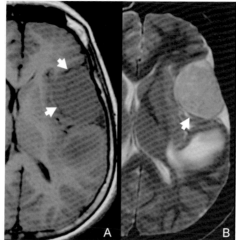

Axial T1- (A) and T2WI (B) show a classic meningioma. Note CSF-vascular "cleft" (arrows), displacement ("buckling") of GW interface. The mass is isointense with gray matter.

- DSA
  - Pial vessels supply periphery
  - Dural vessels supply lesion core
    - "Sunburst" pattern of enlarged dural feeders
    - Prolonged vascular "stain"
- SPECT: High uptake of somatostatin analog

Differential Diagnosis
Dural Metastasis
- Overlying skull often involved
- Breast metastasis may be indistinguishable

Other
- Sarcoid
- Idiopathic hypertrophic pachymeningitis (see "Pachymeningiopathy" diagnosis)
- Dural vascular malformation (e.g., hemangioma)
- Hemangiopericytoma

Pathology
General
- General Path Comments
  - Generally slowly growing, benign tumors
- Genetics
  - Sporadic
    - Up to 60% have NF 2 (chromosome 22) gene mutations
    - Most express GH receptors
    - Progression, anaplasia associated with other allelic losses
  - Multiple
    - NF2 (N.B.: Multiple meningiomatosis can occur without NF2)
    - Monoclonal origin

Meningioma

- Etiology-Pathogenesis-Pathophysiology
  - Dura "tail"
    - Tumor in vascular pedicle at site of attachment
    - Vascular congestion in adjacent dura
    - Thickened dura contains increased loose connective tissue, dilated vessels
    - Usually no tumor invasion
  - Arise from arachnoid meningothelial ("cap") cells
  - Peritumoral edema related to pial blood supply, VEGF expression
- Epidemiology
  - Account for 15%-20% of primary intracranial tumors
  - 1%-1.5% prevalence at autopsy
  - 90% supratentorial (parasagittal/convexity > sphenoid ridge > olfactory groove/planum sphenoidale > juxtasellar)
  - 8%-10% infratentorial (CPA most common)
  - 1%-2% miscellaneous (e.g., intraventricular, paranasal sinus)

Gross Pathologic or Surgical Features
- Well-demarcated round/lobulated or "en plaque" dural-based mass
- Hyperostosis, skull invasion common
- Nonneoplastic dural thickening ("dural tail") common
- Rarely show overt brain invasion

Microscopic Features
- Meningioma has wide range of subtypes
  - Meningothelial (uniform tumor cells, collagenous septa)
  - Fibrous (interlacing fascicles of spindle-shaped cells, collagen/ reticulin matrix)
  - Transitional (mixed; "onion-bulb" whorls, psammoma bodies)
  - Others = angiomatous (**not** to be confused with hemangiopericytoma), microcystic, secretory, chordoid,etc
- Atypical meningioma (increased mitoses, cellularity, etc.)
- Anaplastic (malignant) meningioma

Staging or Grading Criteria
- 90% are WHO grade I
- 5%-7% = WHO grade II (atypical, clear cell, chordoid)
- 1%-3% = WHO grade III (anaplastic, rhabdoid, papillary, invasive)

Clinical Issues

Presentation
- Middle-aged, elderly patients (35-70y) but can occur in children
- Female: Male = 2:1
- Symptoms location dependent; 1/3 asymptomatic

Natural History
- Generally grow slowly, compress adjacent structures

Treatment & Prognosis
- Incompletely resected, atypical/anaplastic meningiomas, tumors with high VEGF expression have higher recurrence rate

Selected References
1. Filippi CG et al: Appearance of meningiomas on DWI: Correlating diffusion constants with histopathologic findings. AJNR 22:65-72, 2001
2. Kawahara Y et al: Dural congestion accompanying meningioma invasion into vessels: the dural tail sign. Neuroradiol 43: 462-65, 2001
3. Louis DN et al: Meningiomas. In Kleihues P, Cavenee WK (eds), Tumours of the Nervous System, 176-84, IARC Press, 2000

Hemangioblastoma

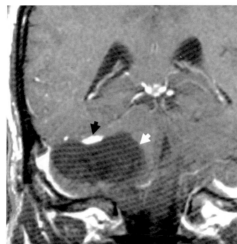

Coronal contrast-enhanced T1WI shows a cystic cerebellar mass (white arrow). Strongly-enhancing nodule (black arrow) abuts the pia. Sporadic hemangioblastoma.

Key Facts
- Most common posterior fossa intra-axial mass in middle-aged/older adult = metastasis, **not** hemangioblastoma (HGB)
- 75% of HGBs are sporadic; 25% occur with von Hippel-Lindau (VHL) disease

Imaging Findings
General Features
- See "VHL" diagnosis
- 60% cyst + "mural" nodule; 40% solid
- Best diagnostic sign= cystic mass with enhancing mural nodule abutting pia

CT Findings
- NECT: Low density cyst + isodense nodule
- CECT
  - Common: Nodule enhances strongly, uniformly; cyst doesn't
  - Less common: Solid tumor
  - Rare: Ring enhancing mass

MR Findings
- Sensitivity of MR >> CT for small HGBs
- Cyst hypo-, nodule isointense with brain on T1WI
- Hyperintense on T2WI
- Prominent "flow voids" in some cases
- Nodule enhances strongly, intensely

Other Modality Findings
- DSA: Large avascular mass (cyst) + highly vascular nodule (prolonged blush, sometimes A-V shunting)
- Thallium-201 SPECT shows fast washout

Imaging Recommendations
- Begin MRI screening of patients from VHL families after age 10y

Hemangioblastoma

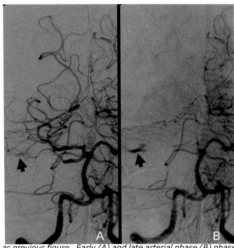

Same case as previous figure. Early (A) and late arterial phase (B) phase of vertebral angiogram shows the tumor nodule has a vascular blush (arrow). Hemangioblastoma.

Differential Diagnosis

<u>Metastasis</u>
- Most common parenchymal posterior fossa mass in middle-aged, older adults
- Usually not as vascular as HGB

<u>Glioma</u>
- Very rare posterior fossa mass in older adults

<u>Other</u>
- Clear cell ependymoma

Pathology

<u>General</u>
- General Path Comments
  - VHL phenotypes
    - Type 1 = without pheochromocytoma
    - Type 2A = with pheochromocytoma, renal cell carcinoma (RCC)
    - Type 2B = with pheochromocytoma, without RCC
- Genetics
  - Familial HGB (VHL disease)
    - Autosomal dominant
    - Chromosome 3p mutation
    - Suppressor gene product (VHL protein) causes neoplastic transformation
    - VEGF highly expressed in stromal cells
    - Other VHL gene mutations common
  - Sporadic HGB
    - Upregulation of erythropoietin common in both sporadic, VHL-related HGB
- Etiology-Pathogenesis-Pathophysiology
  - Unknown origin

Hemangioblastoma

- Epidemiology
  - 2% of primary CNS tumors
    - 7%-10% of posterior fossa tumors
    - Rare: Supratentorial (usually along optic pathways)
  - 3%-13% of spinal cord tumors
  - 75% of HGB are sporadic; 25% associated with VHL

Gross Pathologic or Surgical Features
- Well-circumscribed, highly vascular nodule +/- cyst

Microscopic Features
- Cyst wall usually compressed brain, not neoplasm
- Nodule = large, vacuolated stromal cells + rich capillary network

Staging or Grading Criteria
- WHO grade I

Clinical Issues

Presentation
- Sporadic HGB
  - 40-60 y
  - Headache (85%), dysequilibrium, dizziness
- Familial
  - VHL-associated HGBs occur at younger age but are rare < 15y
  - Retinal HGB
    - Ocular hemorrhage often first manifestation of VHL
    - Mean onset 25y
  - Other: Sx due to RCC, polycythemia, endolymphatic sac tumor

Natural History
- Benign tumor with slow growth pattern
- Two-thirds with one VHL-associated HGB develop additional lesions
  - Average = one new lesion every 2 years
  - Require period screening, lifelong follow-up

Treatment & Prognosis
- Surgical resection +/- pre-operative embolization
  - 85% 10 year survival rate
  - 15%-20% recurrence rate
  - Median life expectancy in VHL = 49 years

Selected References
1. Conway JE et al: Hemangioblastomas of the CNS in von Hippel-Lindau syndrome and sporadic disease. Neurosurg 48: 55-63, 2001
2. Kondo T et al: Diagnostic value of 201Tl-single-photon emission computerized tomography studies in cases of posterior fossa hemangioblastomas. J Neurosurg 95: 292-7, 2001
3. Bohling T et al: von Hippel-Lindau disease and capillary hemangioblastoma. In Kleihues P, Cavenee WK (eds): Tumours of the Nervous System, 223-6, IARC Press, 2000

Medulloblastoma (PNET-MB)

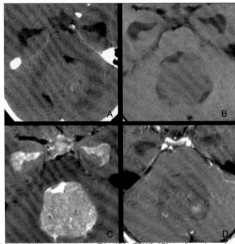

Axial CECT scan (A), pre-contrast T1- (B), T2WI (C) and post-contrast T1WI (D) show a medulloblastoma (PNET-MB). The mass fills the fourth ventricle, shows minimal patchy enhancement.

Key Facts
- Medulloblastoma = posterior fossa PNET (PNET-MB)
- Malignant, invasive, highly cellular embryonal tumor of the cerebellum (vermis)
- Most common childhood posterior fossa tumor in some series
- Midline >> off-midline
- Inherent tendency for CSF metastasis

Imaging Findings
General Features
- Best diagnostic sign = round, high-density, midline posterior fossa mass (looks like baseball stuck inside 4th ventricle)
- Off-midline location increases with age

CT Findings
- NECT
  - Hyperdense, mostly solid, midline posterior fossa mass
  - Less common: Isodense, inhomogeneous (cysts)
  - 10%-20% Ca++
  - 4th ventricle displaced anteriorly, draped over mass
  - Hydrocephalus common (95%)
- CECT
  - > 90% enhance
    - Degree varies from mild to moderate
    - Pattern varies from patchy to relatively uniform

MR Findings
- Usually homogeneous midline (4th ventricle) mass
  - Iso-/hypointense to GM on T1WI
  - Isointense on T2WI; may be mixed hyper/hypo-
  - +/- Cyst, hemorrhage, necrosis
- 90% variable enhancement
- 50% CSF spread at initial imaging

Medulloblastoma (PNET-MB)

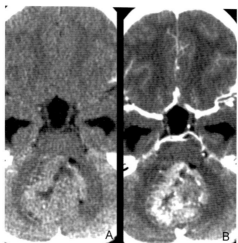

NECT (A) and CECT (B) scans of typical medulloblastoma (PNET- MB). Note "baseball" appearance of high-density mass in 4th ventricle.

Other Modality Findings
- MRS: Low NAA:Cho, Cr:Cho ratios

Imaging Recommendations
- Image entire neuraxis before surgery for CSF spread

Differential Diagnosis

Pilocytic Astrocytoma
- Hypodense on NECT
- Often off midline
- Cyst with mural nodule> solid

Ependymoma
- "Plastic" tumor within fourth ventricle, extrudes through foramina
- Ca++, cysts, hemorrhage common
- Heterogeneous enhancement

Brainstem Glioma
- Hypodense (often dorsally exophytic) brainstem mass
- Displaces 4th ventricle posteriorly
- Minimal/no enhancement

Pathology

General
- General Path Comments
  - Medulloblastoma = most common embryonal tumor subtype
  - Location
    - 75% arise in cerebellar vermis
    - Off-midline location (cerebellum) increases with age, more common with desmoplastic variant
- Genetics
  - Syndromic PNET-MBs
    - Nevoid basal cell carcinoma (Gorlin) syndrome (2% of PNET-MBs; look for falx Ca++)

Medulloblastoma (PNET-MB)

- - Turcot syndrome (polyposis coli+ MB/malignant gliomas)
    - Li-Fraumeni syndrome (TP53 germline mutation)
  - o Solitary: 50% have isochromosome 17q abnormalities
- Etiology-Pathogenesis (three hypotheses)
  - o Originate from external granular layer of cerebellum
  - o Derive from subependymal matrix cells (precursor cell)
  - o More than one cell of origin (ventricular matrix & external granular layer)
- Epidemiology
  - o 15-20% of intracranial tumors in children
  - o Bimodal age distribution
    - Most MBs occur in childhood (mean age = 7y)
    - Second, smaller peak in adults (21-40y)
  - o M:F = approximately 2:1
  - o MB = most common tumor to metastasize outside CNS (bone)

Gross Pathologic or Surgical Features
- Variable (ranges from firm/discrete to soft/less well defined)

Microscopic Features
- Densely packed cells, round-to-oval nuclei, scant cytoplasm
- Poorly-differentiated (primitive) neuroepithelial cells
- Neuroblastic rosettes typical (Homer Wright)
- Mitoses and apoptosis frequent
- Hypercellular tumor with high nuclear:cytoplasmic ratio
- 4 subtypes
  - o Desmoplastic MB
  - o MB with extensive nodularity
  - o Large cell MB
  - o Melanotic MB
- Immunohistochemistry: +/- Synaptophysin, vimentin, GFAP etc.

Staging or Grading Criteria
- WHO grade IV

Clinical Issues

Presentation
- Truncal ataxia, disturbed gait, lethargy
- Headache, vomiting (obstructive hydrocephalus)

Natural History
- Early CSF dissemination (up to 50% at initial presentation)

Treatment & Prognosis
- Surgical resection, focal XRT (>50Gy); 25- 45Gy to remainder of brain and spine in pts > 3y
- Adjuvant chemotherapy
- 5-year survival 50-80%
- Poor risk = Age < 3y, CSF dissemination at presentation, incomplete resection

Selected References
1. Giangaspero F et al: Medulloblastoma. In Kleihues P, Cavenee WK (eds), Pathology & Genetics of Tumours of the Nervous System, 129-37, 2000
2. Meyers SP et al: Postoperative evaluation for disseminated medulloblastoma involving the spine: contrast-enhanced MR Findings, CSF cytologic analysis, timing of disease occurrence, and patient outcomes. Am J Neuroradiol 21:1757-65, 2000
3. Stavrou T et al: Intracranial calcifications in childhood medulloblastoma: Relation to nevoid basal cell carcinoma syndrome. AFNR 21: 790-4, 2000

Primary CNS Lymphoma

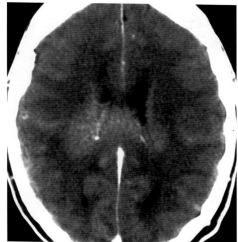

Axial post-contrast CT scan shows a mildly enhancing corpus callosum mass. Primary CNS lymphoma.

Key Facts
- Incidence increasing in immunocompetent, immunocompromised
- Vast majority NHL (B-cell lymphoma)
- Enhancing lesion(s) within basal ganglia, periventricular WM
- Imaging and prognosis varies with immune status

Imaging Findings
General Features
- Lesions cluster around ventricles, GM-WM junction
- Often involve, cross corpus callosum
- Frequently abut, extend along ependymal surfaces
- Best diagnostic sign = periventricular/basal ganglia mass with density/intensity like GM

CT Findings
- NECT
  - Hyperdense, occasionally isodense
  - +/- Hemorrhage, necrosis (immunocompromised)
- CECT
  - Common: Moderate, uniform (immunocompetent)
  - Less common: Ring (immunocompromised)
  - Rare: Nonenhancing (infiltrative, mimics white matter disease)

MR Findings
- Signal like gray matter (varies if hemorrhage, necrosis)
  - Iso/hypointense to cortex on both T1-, T2WI
  - FLAIR usually hyperintense
- Strong homogeneous enhancement (immunocompetent)

Other Modality Findings
- DWI: Restricted diffusion, low ADC map reported
- MRS: NAA decreased, Cho elevated; + lip/lac peaks reported

Imaging Recommendations
- See "HIV" diagnosis

Primary CNS Lymphoma

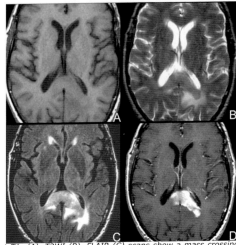

Pre-contrast T1- (A), T2WI (B), FLAIR (C) scans show a mass crossing the corpus callosum splenium. The lesion is mostly isointense with gray matter. (D) Post-contrast T1WI shows strong uniform enhancement. Primary CNS lymphoma.

Differential Diagnosis
Toxoplasmosis
- Often indistinguishable on standard MRI
  - Hyperintense on DWI
  - SPECT, PET helpful
- May hemorrhage after treatment
- Subependymal spread suggests lymphoma
- Solitary subependymal lesion in HIV+ patient usually lymphoma

Glioblastoma Multiforme ("Butterfly Glioma")
- Hemorrhage common
- Necrosis with ring enhancement in 95%

Sarcoid
- Dural, leptomeningeal >> parenchymal disease
- Most patients have systemic disease

White Matter Disease
- May be indistinguishable
- Enhancement uncommon

Secondary Involvement From Systemic Lymphoma
- Intravascular pattern common
- Can have single/multiple deep, periventricular lesions

Pathology
General
- General Path Comments
  - 98% B cell lymphoma; rarely T-cell
  - 90% supratentorial; circumscribed > infiltrative pattern
  - Multiple lesions in 20%-25% (usually immunocompromised)
- Etiology-Pathogenesis
  - Inherited or acquired immunodeficiency predisposes

- o EBV plays major role in immunocompromised
- Epidemiology
  - o 1%-7% of primary brain tumors, rising

Gross Pathologic or Surgical Features
- Single or multiple masses in cerebral hemispheres
- Central necrosis, hemorrhage in HIV+

Microscopic Features
- Angiocentric (surrounds, infiltrates vessels and perivascular spaces)
- Several subtypes (large cell accounts for nearly 50%)
- High nuclear/cytoplasmic ratio (high electron density)
- Mitoses, labeling indices?

Clinical Issues
Presentation
- All ages
  - o Immunocompetent = 6th – 7th decade
  - o Immunocompromised
    - Inherited immunodeficiency syndromes (mean 10y)
    - Transplant recipients (mean 37y)
    - AIDS (mean 39y)
- Symptoms
  - o Focal neurologic deficit, seizure
  - o Cognitive, neuropsychiatric disturbance
  - o Headache, increased intracranial pressure

Natural History
- Dramatic but short-lived response to steroids/ XRT

Treatment & Prognosis
- Favorable prognostic factors: Single lesion, absence of meningeal or periventricular dz, immunocompetent pt, age < 60 years
- Current Rx: RT & chemo – median survival 17-45 months
- AIDS–median survival 2-6 months / multimodality Rx- 13.5 months

Selected References
1. Stadnik TW et al: Diffusion-weighted MR imaging of intracerebral masses: Comparison with conventional MR imaging and histologic findings. AJNR 22: 969-76, 2001
2. Bataille B et al: Primary intracerebral malignant lymphoma: Report of 248 cases. J Neurosurgery 92:261-6, 2000
3. Paulus W et al: Malignant lymphomas. In Kleihues P, Cavenee WK (eds), Pathology & Genetics of Tumours of the Nervous System, 198-203. IARC Press, 2000

Germinoma

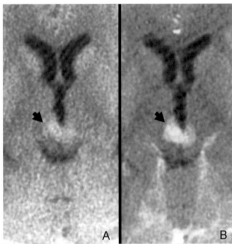

CT scan without (A) and with contrast enhancement (B) shows a high-density, enhancing mass that engulfs the pineal gland, posterior 3rd ventricle, and extends into the thalami (arrows). Germinoma.

Key Facts
- CNS germ cell tumors (GCTs) homologous with gonadal, extragonadal tumors
- Affect mainly children, adolescents
- Germinoma (a.k.a. seminoma, dysgerminoma, formerly called atypical teratoma) = most common type

Imaging Findings
<u>General Features</u>
- Except for teratoma, imaging features of intracranial germ cell tumors nonspecific, often overlap other
  - Most common: Solid mass at posterior 3rd ventricle
- Best diagnostic sign = germinoma "engulfs" calcified pineal gland

<u>CT Findings</u>
- NECT
  - Iso/hyperdense mass draped around posterior 3rd ventricle
  - Surrounds nodular cluster of Ca++ (the "engulfed" pineal gland)
  - Hydrocephalus
- CECT
  - Strong uniform enhancement
  - Look for other lesions (suprasellar, ependymal)

<u>MR Findings</u>
- Usually iso- to slightly hypointense on T1WI
- Hyperintense on T2WI
- Cysts, heterogeneous signal in 75%
- Strong but heterogeneous enhancement
- Multiple lesions in almost 50%

<u>Other Modality Findings</u>
- CSF tumor markers (AFP, ß-HCG) usually negative unless mixed histology

Germinoma

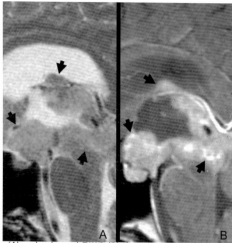

Sagittal T2- (A) and enhanced T1WI (B) demonstrate an extensive mass that is isointense with GM. The lesion involves the pineal and suprasellar regions, pituitary gland and stalk, and ventricles (arrows). Germinoma.

- Isolated elevation of PLAP suggests germinoma

<u>Imaging Recommendations</u>
- MR without, with contrast enhancement
- Scan entire neuraxis for CSF dissemination

Differential Diagnosis
<u>Other GCT</u>
- Teratoma (second most common pineal region tumor)
  - Two or more embryologic layers
  - Usually much more heterogeneous
- Mixed GCT

<u>Pineal Parenchymal Tumor</u>
- Pineoblastoma, pineocytoma

<u>Other Pineal Region Mass</u>
- Meningioma, metastasis
- Infection, inflammation (e.g., sarcoid, TB)

Pathology
<u>General</u>
- General Path Comments
  - Unencapsulated solid mass, may have small cystic foci
  - Necrosis, hemorrhage uncommon unless tumor in basal ganglia
  - Location
    - 80%-90% midline (pineal >> suprasellar > both)
    - 5%-10% basal ganglia, thalamus
- Genetics: At least two classes within GCTs
  - Congenital/infantile teratomas, yolk sac tumors
    - Diploidy
    - Normal chromosome 12 profiles

Germinoma

- o   Peri-, post-pubertal germinomas
  - ▪   Aneuploidy
  - ▪   Overrepresentation of chromosome 12p
- • Etiology-Pathogenesis: Two theories of how intracranial GCTs develop
  - o   Abnormal histogenesis
    - ▪   Embryonic disc gives rise to primary, secondary yolk sac
    - ▪   Primordial germ cells persist
    - ▪   Germ cells maldifferentiate into germinoma
  - o   Aberrant migration ("incorrect involvement and enfoldment")
    - ▪   Cells from yolk sac endoderm (amnion) or trophoblast move toward midline
    - ▪   Cells enter primitive groove
    - ▪   Cells migrate to neural plate
    - ▪   As neural tube folds, cells are incorporated into neuraxis
    - ▪   Germ cell tumors develop later from "misenfolded" cells
- • Epidemiology
  - o   Intracranial GCTs comprise 0.1-3.4% of primary CNS neoplasms
  - o   Germinoma accounts for 2/3rd of all GCTs
  - o   90% affect patients < 20y
    - ▪   Peak age = 10-12y
    - ▪   M:F = 2:1

Gross Pathologic or Surgical Features
- • Soft and friable, tan-white mass

Microscopic Features
- • Sheets/lobules of uniform cells
  - o   Large nuclei
  - o   Prominent nucleoli
  - o   Clear, glycogen-rich cytoplasm (PAS-positive)
- • Lymphocytic infiltrates along fibrovascular septa common
- • May be histologically mixed with other GCTs

Clinical Issues
Presentation
- • HA, visual disturbances, Parinaud syndrome
- • Diabetes insipidus, growth disturbances

Natural History
- • Invades adjacent brain (e.g., thalamus)
- • CSF dissemination common

Treatment & Prognosis
- • Stereotaxic/endoscopic biopsy
- • XRT +/- adjuvant chemotherapy
- • 75%-95% 5 year survival

Selected References
1.   Rosenblum MK et al: CNS germ cell tumors. In Kleihues P, Cavenee WK (eds), Tumours of the Nervous System, 207-14, IARC Press, 2000
2.   Sano K: Pathogenesis of intracranial germ cell tumors reconsidered. J Neurosurg 90: 258-64, 1999
3.   Smirniotopoulos JG et al: Pineal region masses: Differential diagnosis. RadioGraphics 12: 577-96, 1992

Pineal Parenchymal Tumors

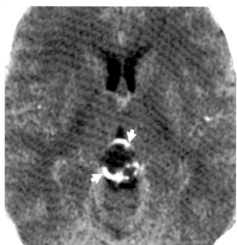

CECT scan shows a 15 mm posterior third ventricular mass that "explodes" the calcified pineal gland (arrows). Pineocytoma.

Key Facts
- Pineal parenchymal tumors << germinoma
- Tumors derive from pinealocytes/embryonal precursors
- Two major types: Highly malignant, primitive pineoblastoma (PB) and mature pineocytoma (PC)

Imaging Findings
General Features
- Best diagnostic sign = "exploded" pineal (vs. "engulfed" with germinoma)

CT Findings
- PB: Mixed density, weak to moderate heterogeneous enhancement, peripheral Ca++ common
- PC: Mass iso/hypodense to brain, peripheral Ca++

MR Findings
- PB: Irregular, poorly-delineated mass
  - Iso/hypo on T1-, hyperintense on T2WI
  - Moderate heterogeneous enhancement
  - Invades corpus callosum, thalamus, midbrain
- PC: Well-delineated, round/lobulated mass
  - Iso/hypo on T1-, hyperintense on T2WI
  - Strong enhancement (homogeneous solid ring)
  - Compresses tectum

Other Modality Findings
- PB, PC negative for α-fetoprotein, HCG

Imaging Recommendations
- Suspected PB, germinoma, etc.): Image entire neuraxis
- PC (see Pineal Cyst diagnosis)

Pineal Parenchymal Tumors

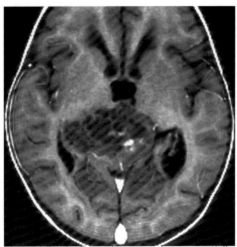

Contrast-enhanced T1WI of pineoblastoma shows a partially enhancing inhomogeneous mass at the pineal/posterior third ventricular region.

Differential Diagnosis

Nonneoplastic Pineal (Glial) Cyst
- See "Pineal Cyst" diagnosis
- May be indistinguishable from PC on imaging studies

Neoplasm
- Germinoma
- Other pineal region neoplasm (astrocytoma, meningioma, etc.)

Pathology

General
- General Path Comments
  - Pineal parenchymal tumors can show retinoblastomatous, astrocytic, neuronal or mixed differentiation
  - Span wide spectrum from neoplasm with mature elements (PC) to primitive immature cells (PB)
  - PBs are similar to other PNETs
- Genetics
  - No TP53 mutations
  - Some reports of chromosome 11 deletions in PBs
  - "Trilateral retinoblastoma" has bilateral RBs, pineal PNET like PB
- Etiology-Pathogenesis-Pathophysiology
  - Derived from pineal parenchymal cells ("pinealocytes") or their embryonic precursors
  - Pinealocytes = cells with photosensory, neuroendocrine function
- Epidemiology
  - 0.5%-1% of primary brain tumors
  - 15% of pineal region neoplasms

Gross Pathologic or Surgical Features
- PB = soft, friable, poorly marginated (infiltrates adjacent tissues)
- PC = well-circumscribed, gray-tan mass (may compress but doesn't invade adjacent structures)

Pineal Parenchymal Tumors

Microscopic Features
- PB = highly cellular tumor
  - Sheets of densely packed, small, undifferentiated cells
  - Round, carrot-shaped hyperchromatic nuclei, scanty cytoplasm
  - Occasional Homer-Wright or Flexner-Wintersteiner rosettes
  - Immunolabeling for synaptophysin, neuronal specific enolase (NSE) + but lower compared to PCs, mixed tumors
  - Necrosis in majority of cases
  - Mitoses common, MIB1 elevated
- PC
  - Sheets or lobules of tumor separated by mesenchymal septa
  - Small, uniform, mature cells resemble pinealocytes
  - Large fibrillary "pinocytomatous rosettes"
  - Cysts, hemorrhage not infrequent
  - Mitoses, necrosis absent
  - Stains intensely for synaptophysin, NSE
  - Can be pleomorphic with mixed/intermediate differentiation, mitoses, occasional areas of necrosis, endothelial hyperplasia

Staging or Grading Criteria
- WHO
  - PB = grade IV
  - PC = grade II
- New
  - Grade 1 for PC
  - Grade 2 if < 6 mitoses
  - Grade 3 with =>6 mitoses or <6 mitoses but without immunostaining for neurofilaments
  - Grade 4 for PB

Clinical Issues
Presentation
- Like other pineal region masses (see "Pineal Cysts," "Germinoma")

Natural History
- PB = Metastasizes (CNS, bone)
- PC = Stable/slow growing

Treatment & Prognosis
- Stereotactic biopsy, ventriculoscopy
- PB = 0% (grade 4) to 40% (grade 3) 5 year survival
- PC = 90% (grade 2) to 100% (grade 1) 5 year survival

Selected References
1. Fauchon F et al: Parenchymal pineal tumors: A clinicopathological study of 76 cases. Int J Rad Onc Biol Phys 4: 959-68, 2000
2. Nakamura M et al: Neuroradiological characteristics of pineocytoma and pineoblastoma. Neuroradiol 42: 509-14, 2000
3. Jouvet A et al: Pineal parenchymal tumors: A correlation of histological features with prognosis in 66 cases. Brain Pathol 10: 49-60, 2000

Schwannoma

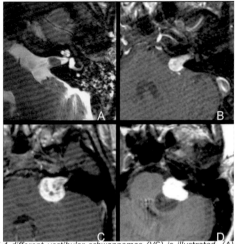

A series of 4 different vestibular schwannomas (VS) is illustrated. (A) Axial T2WI shows a small intracanalicular VS. (B) Contrast-enhanced T1WI shows the classic "ice cream on a cone" appearance of VS projecting into the CPA. (C) A larger, more inhomogeneous VS is shown. (D) VS with an associated cyst.

Key Facts
- Second most common intracranial extra-axial neoplasm in adults
- 90% arise from CN VIII
- Vestibular schwannoma (VS) = most common CPA/IAC mass

Imaging Findings
General Features
- Slow-growing extra-axial mass
  - Displaces ("buckles") cortex
  - CSF-vascular "cleft" between tumor, brain
- Best diagnostic sign: VS looks like "ice cream on cone"

CT Findings
- NECT
  - Noncalcified CPA mass
  - Iso/slightly hyperdense compared to brain
  - May enlarge IAC
- CECT
  - Strong, uniform enhancement

MR Findings
- Usually iso-, sometimes mixed iso-/hypointense on T1WI
  - 15% intratumoral cysts (occasionally have fluid-fluid level)
  - 2% associated arachnoid cyst
  - 1% hemorrhage
- > 95% hyperintense on T2WI
- Enhances strongly
  - 2/3 solid; 1/3 ring or inhomogeneous

Other Modality Findings
- DSA
  - Hypovascular mass (adjacent vessels stretched, draped)
  - Diffuse blush, AV shunting rare

Schwannoma

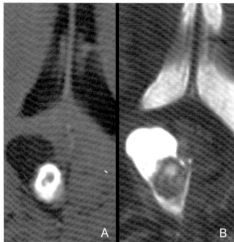

Axial post-contrast T1- (A), T2WI (B) show a cortically-based mass with well-delineated cyst and enhancing nodule. Intraparenchymal schwannoma was found at surgery (courtesy J. Rees).

Imaging Recommendations
- High-resolution screening MRI of temporal bones/CPA for SNHL

Differential Diagnosis
Meningioma
- Broad dural base, usually doesn't extend into IAC
- May cause hyperostosis
- Dural "tail" common (rare: VS may have reactive dural thickening)
- Usually isointense with cortex on T2WI (schwannoma hyperintense)
- Rare: Purely intracanalicular meningioma can mimic small VS
Other Schwannoma
- CN VII schwannoma confined to CPA may mimic VS
- CN V schwannoma often involves Meckel's cave
Epidermoid or Arachnoid Cyst vs. Cystic VS
- No enhancement
Metastasis
- Bone destruction common
- Known primary
Other
- MPNST: Rare; most reported cases after XRT
- Hemangioma

Pathology
General
- General Path Comments
  - Involve sensory > motor nerves; 1% intraparenchymal
- Genetics
  - Solitary
    - Loss of Merlin expression
    - Inactivating mutations of NF2 gene in 60%

Schwannoma

- - Loss of remaining wild-type allele on chromosome 22q
  - o Multiple: NF2 (see "NF2"), less often multiple schwannomatosis (without NF-2 stigmata)
- Epidemiology
  - o 8% of primary intracranial neoplasms

Gross Pathologic or Surgical Features
- Tan, round/ovoid, encapsulated extra-axial mass
- May have bright yellow patches, hemorrhage
- 15%-20% associated cysts (intralesional or peritumoral)

Microscopic Features
- Spindle-shaped neoplastic Schwann cells
- Arises at glial-Schwann cell junction (VS = near porus acousticus)
- Two types of intermixed tissue
  - o Antoni A (compact, elongated cells, +/- nuclear palisading)
  - o Antoni B (less cellular, loosely textured, often lipidized)
- Other variants = melanotic schwannoma

Staging or Grading Criteria
- WHO grade I

Clinical Issues
Presentation
- Varies depending on cranial/spinal nerve involved
- VS: Tinnitus, sensorineural hearing loss, facial paresthesias

Natural History
- Slowly growing; recurrence after surgery < 10%
- Factors associated with growth = tumors with cysts, no IAC component, females, younger patients
- Malignant degeneration exceptionally rare

Treatment & Prognosis
- Microsurgical resection
  - o 90% normal/near-normal CN VII function (VS removal)
  - o 40% hearing preservation
- Stereotactic radiosurgery
- Some smaller tumors/older patients managed with observation

Selected References
1. Nutik SL et al: Determinants of tumor size and growth in vestibular schwannomas. J Neurosurg 94: 922-6, 2001
2. Woodruff JM et al: Schwannoma. In Kleihues P, Cavenee WK (eds), Tumours of the Nervous System, 164-6, IARC Press, 2000
3. Sampath P et al: Microanatomical variations in the cerebellopontine angle associated with vestibular schwannomas (acoustic neuromas). J Neurosurg 92: 70-8, 2000

Neurofibroma (NF)

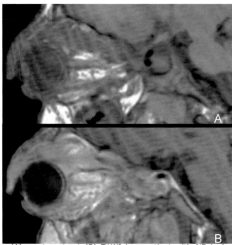

Sagittal pre- (A), post-contrast (B) T1WI in a patient with NF-1 show an orbital plexiform neurofibroma that extends posteriorly through an expanded superior orbital fissure into the cavernous sinus (courtesy B. Haas).

Key Facts
- NFs may affect spinal roots, rarely cranial nerves
- Can be sporadic, associated with NF-1
- Plexiform neurofibroma is hallmark of NF-1
- Orbit is most common site in head/neck

Imaging Findings
General Features
- Can be well-demarcated (solitary NF) or diffusely infiltrating (plexiform NF)
- Best diagnostic sign = "wormlike" infiltrating soft-tissue mass in patient with NF-1
CT Findings
- Solitary: Isodense, strongly-enhancing nodular mass
- Plexiform
  - Mass infiltrates CN V_1
  - May extend through orbital fissure into cavernous sinus but almost never posterior to Meckel's cave
- Other sites: Scalp, skull base
MR Findings
- Plexiform NF
  - Multilobulated insinuating mass
  - Iso- on T1-, hyperintense on T2WI
  - Moderate enhancement
Imaging Recommendations
- MR without and with contrast
- CT (bone algorithm) if plexiform NF at skull base

Neurofibroma (NF)

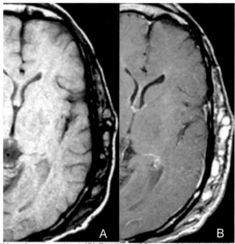

Axial pre- (A) and post-contrast (B) T1WI in a 23-year-old patient with known NF-1 show an extensive plexiform neurofibroma infiltrating the scalp.

Differential Diagnosis

Schwannoma
- Usually solitary, well-circumscribed
- May involve CNs, spinal nerve roots

Malignant Peripheral Nerve Sheath Tumor (MPNST)
- 50% occur in setting of NF-1
- Diffusely infiltrating, may invade bone

Pathology

General
- General Path Comments
  - Can be focal, well-demarcated or diffuse/ infiltrating
- Genetics
  - NF-1 associated NFs
    - Germline NF-1 mutation
    - Loss of remaining wild-type allele
    - Monoclonal
  - Sporadic NF: Unknown
- Etiology-Pathogenesis-Pathophysiology
  - "Two-hits" hypothesis for genesis of NFs
- Epidemiology
  - All ages, both sexes
  - Multiple NFs are hallmark of NF-1
  - Plexiform NF is pathognomonic for NF-1

Gross Pathologic or Surgical Features
- Plexiform NF
  - Infiltrating poorly-delineated mass
  - Looks like "bag of worms"
  - Often involves multiple nerve fascicles

- Solitary NF (e.g., spinal nerve root)
  - Firm, well-circumscribed intraneural nodule
  - Grayish-tan, ovoid/fusiform

Microscopic Features
- Neoplastic Schwann cells
- Fibroblasts
- Matrix of collagen fibers, mucoid substances
- Stains + for S-100 protein

Staging or Grading Criteria
- NF = WHO grade I
- MPNST= WHO grade III or IV

Clinical Issues

Presentation
- Painless mass
  - Cutaneous nodule
  - Circumscribed peripheral nerve mass
  - Plexiform enlargement of nerve trunk
- Cranial nerve involvement
  - Orbit, cavernous sinus (CN V) = most common site in head/neck for plexiform NF
  - Less common = CN VII
  - Involvement of other CNs almost unknown
- Spinal nerve NF may cause sciatica
- Look for other stigmata of NF-1 (café-au-lait spots, axillary freckling, Lisch nodules, etc.)

Natural History
- Slow growth
- 2%-12% of plexiform NFs, NFs of major nerves degenerate into malignant peripheral nerve sheath tumor (MPNST)

Treatment & Prognosis
- +/- Surgical resection
- High recurrence rate for plexiform NF

Selected References
1. Woodruff JM et al: Neurofibroma. In Kleihues P, Cavenee WK (eds), Tumours of the Nervous System, 167-8, IARC Press, 2000
2. Needle MN et al: Prognostic signs in the surgical management of plexiform neurofibroma. J Pediatr 131: 678-82, 1997
3. Webber JT et al: Orbital plexiform neurofibroma. IJNR 1: 102-8, 1995

Pituitary Macroadenoma

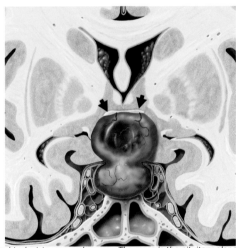

Coronal graphic depicts macroadenoma. The mass is the pituitary gland and cannot be separated from it. Note "figure-of-eight" appearance as the adenoma bulges upwards through the diaphragma sellae. The optic chiasm (arrows) is thinned, draped over the mass.

Key Facts
- Upward extension of macroadenoma = most common suprasellar mass in adults
- "Giant" macroadenomas may be extremely invasive, mimic metastasis, other malignant neoplasms

Imaging Findings
General Features
- Lobulated "figure-of-eight" or "snowman" appearance
- Best diagnostic sign = no identifiable pituitary gland; mass **is** the gland
CT Findings
- NECT
  - Variable; usually isodense with GM
  - Cyst formation, necrosis common
  - Hemorrhage 10%, Ca++ 1%-2%
  - Large adenomas expand sella, may erode floor
  - Aggressive adenomas extend inferiorly, invade sphenoid
- CECT
  - Moderate, somewhat inhomogeneous enhancement
MR Findings
- Usually isointense with GM on all sequences
  - Subacute hemorrhage has short T1
  - Fluid-fluid levels may occur, especially with pituitary apoplexy
- Almost all macroadenomas enhance
  - Early, intense but heterogeneous
  - Mild/moderate dural thickening ("tail") often present
- Cavernous sinus invasion (difficult to determine with certainty)
  - Medial wall of cavernous sinus is thin, weak
  - Benign, nonaggressive adenoma often extend into cavernous sinus
    - ICA encasement >2/3

Pituitary Macroadenoma

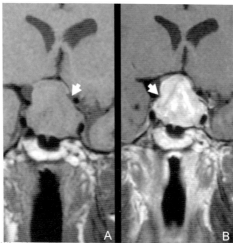

*Coronal T1WI without (A) and with contrast (B) show typical macroadenoma with "figure of eight" appearance (arrows). The macroadenoma **is** the pituitary gland.*

- Occasionally ICA completely encircled
- Asymmetric tentorial enhancement suggests cavernous sinus compression / invasion
- Cannot distinguish invasive but benign adenoma from pituitary carcinoma (exceedingly rare)

Other Modality Findings
- Cavernous/inferior petrosal sinus sampling may be helpful in evaluating ACTH-dependent Cushing syndrome

Imaging Recommendations
- MR without, with contrast (dynamic sequences may be helpful)

Differential Diagnosis

Physiologic Hyperplasia
- 25%-50% of females 18-35y have upwardly convex pituitary
  - Usually< 10 mm unless pregnant, lactating
  - Homogeneous enhancement
  - Normal pituitary function
- Can occur with end-organ failure (e.g., ovarian, thyroid)
- If prepubescent female or young male has "adenoma-looking" pituitary, do endocrine workup!

Aneurysm
- Usually eccentric, not directly suprasellar
- Pituitary gland visible, identified separate from mass
- "Flow void" common on MR
- Ca++ more common

Meningioma (Diaphragma Sellae)
- Pituitary gland visible, identified separate from mass
  - Diaphragma sellae almost always identifiable as thin, dark line between mass (above) and pituitary gland (below)
- Dural thickening more extensive than with adenoma

Malignant Neoplasm (SCCa, Metastasis)
- Diffuse skull base invasion by adenoma may mimic more ominous disease
  - Measure prolactin levels!

Pathology
General
- General Path Comments
  - Usual growth pattern = bulges upward into suprasellar cistern
  - Cavernous sinus invasion at surgery/autopsy in 5%-10%
- Genetics
  - Allelic loss of chromosome 11q in MEN1 region
  - MEN1 gene (probably tumor suppressor) involved in adenoma formation
- Etiology-Pathogenesis
  - See "Microadenoma"
- Epidemiology
  - See "Microadenoma"

Gross Pathologic or Surgical Features
- Reddish-brown, lobulated mass

Microscopic Features
- See "Microadenoma"
- Microscopic dural invasion occurs with most macroadenomas

Staging or Grading Criteria
- WHO grade I
- MIB > 1% suggests early recurrence, rapid regrowth

Clinical Issues
Presentation
- 75% of macroadenomas are endocrinologically active; symptoms vary with adenoma type
- 20-25% visual defect/other cranial nerve palsy
- Pituitary apoplexy (hemorrhagic tumor infarction)
  - Rare but life-threatening, potentially fatal
  - Sudden onset of HA, vomiting, visual symptoms
  - Consciousness disturbances
  - Autonomic or hormonal dysfunction

Natural History
- Benign, slow-growing; malignant transformation rare
- Distant intracranial metastases occur but are exceedingly rare
- Some adenomas (e.g., clinically silent corticotroph adenomas) behave in more aggressive manner with high recurrence rate

Treatment & Prognosis
- Resection (15% recurrence at 8y, 35% at 20 years)
- Other: Medical, stereotaxic radiosurgery, conventional XRT

Selected References
1. Nakasu Y et al: Tentorial enhancement on MR images is a sign of cavernous sinus involvement in patients with sella tumors. AJNR 22: 1528-33,2001
2. Chanson P et al: Normal pituitary hypertrophy as a frequent cause of pituitary incidentaloma: A follow-up study. J Clin Endocrinol Metab 86: 3009-15, 2001
3. Yokoyama S et al: Are nonfunctioning pituitary adnomas extending into the cavernous sinus aggressive and/ or invasive? Neurosurg, Oct 2001 (in press)

Pituitary Microadenoma

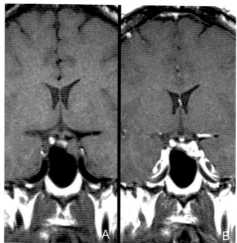

Pre- (A), post-contrast T1WI (B) in a 28 year old female with galactorrhea show a possible mass in the left side of the pituitary gland.

Key Facts
- Microadenomas are 10 mm or less in diameter
- Found incidentally in 10%-20% of autopsies, MR scans
- Pathologically, microadenoma >>> macroadenoma

Imaging Findings
General Features
- Well-demarcated from remainder of pituitary
- Best diagnostic sign = intrapituitary lesion enhancing less rapidly than normal gland

CT Findings
- NECT
  - If uncomplicated (no hemorrhage, cyst), microadenomas are isodense, invisible
- CECT
  - Slow enhancement pattern
  - 2/3rds of microadenomas appear hypodense to normal pituitary on dynamic scans

MR Findings
- Can be hypo-/iso-/hyperintense to normal pituitary gland
- 70-90% identified with T1-/T2-/contrast-enhanced T1WI
- 10%-30% seen only on dynamic contrast-enhanced scans

Other Imaging Findings
- Cavernous/inferior petrosal sinus sampling (10% false negative)

Imaging Recommendations
- Dynamic contrast-enhanced MR

Differential Diagnosis
Nonneoplastic Cyst (Rathke Cleft, Pars Intermedia)
- Endocrine profile usually normal
- Hypo-/hyperintense to normal gland on T1-, T2WI

Pituitary Microadenoma

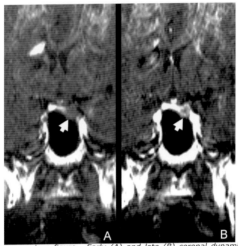

Same case as previous figure. Early (A) and late (B) coronal dynamic contrast-enhanced scans show a focal intrapituitary mass (arrows) with delayed enhancement. Microadenoma.

- No enhancement

<u>Intrasellar Craniopharyngioma</u>
- Uncommon
- May have Ca++
- Displaces normal pituitary
- Enhances (solid, nodular, rim)

Pathology
<u>General</u>
- General Path Comments
  - ○ Common incidental finding at autopsy
  - ○ 10% multiple
- Genetics
  - ○ Clonal origin of pituitary adenomas has been demonstrated
  - ○ No consistent allelic losses or point mutations identified
  - ○ Pituitary tumors can occur as part of MEN1, Carney complex
- Etiology-Pathogenesis
  - ○ One possible model of pituitary tumorigenesis
    - ▪ Hypophysiotrophic hormone excess, suppressive hormone insufficiency, or growth factor excess leads to hyperplasia
    - ▪ Increased proliferation predisposes to genomic instability
    - ▪ Adenoma forms
  - ○ Five endocrine cell types in anterior pituitary (each secretes specific hormone, may develop into micro- or macroadenoma)
    - ▪ Actotrophs = prolactin (PRL)
    - ▪ Somatotrophs = growth hormone (GH)
    - ▪ Corticotrophs = adrenocorticotrophic hormone (ACTH)
    - ▪ Thyrotrophs = thyroid-stimulating hormone (TSH)
    - ▪ Gonadotrophs = gonadotropins, luteinizing hormone, follicle-stimulating hormone

Pituitary Microadenoma

- ○ Excess releasing hormones may also promote growth of genetically transformed cells
- Epidemiology
  - ○ 10%-15% of intracranial tumors
  - ○ Most microadenomas found incidentally at imaging, autopsy (sometimes termed "pituitary incidentaloma")
  - ○ Prolactin-secreting = 30-40% of symptomatic adenomas

Gross Pathologic or Surgical Features
- Small reddish-pink nodule

Microscopic Features
- Monotonous sheets of uniform cells
- Cell type identified with immunohistochemical stains

Staging or Grading Criteria
- Almost always nonmalignant (pituitary carcinoma exceedingly rare)
- Classified according to size
  - ○ Microadenoma = 10 mm or smaller
  - ○ Macroadenoma = > 10 mm

Clinical Issues

Presentation
- Asymptomatic/nonfunctioning
- Symptoms of secreting tumors vary according to type
  - ○ Hyperprolactinemia (most common microadenoma)
    - ▪ Amenorrhea, galactorrhea, infertility
    - ▪ Can also occur with nonprolactin-secreting tumors ("stalk-section effect," "macroprolactinemia" with "big big prolactin")
- Noninvasive laboratory tests (dexamethasone suppression, metyrapone stimulation, peripheral ovine CRH stimulation)

Natural History
- Benign, slow-growing; many never become symptomatic

Treatment & Prognosis
- "Incidentaloma": Conservative (clinical, imaging follow-up unless change in size, ophthalmological/endocrinological evaluation)
- Functioning microadenomas
  - ○ Medical (bromocriptine) reduces PRL secretion to normal in 80%
  - ○ Surgical (rhinoseptal) curative in 60%-90%

Selected References
1. Ezzat S: The role of hormones, growth factors and their receptors in pituitary tumorigenesis. Brain Pathol 11: 356-70, 2001
2. Nishizawa S et al: Therapeutic strategy for incidentally found pituitary tumors ("pituitary incidentalomas"). Neurosurg 43: 1344-50, 1998
3. Bartynski WS et al: Dynamic and conventional spin-echo MR of pituitary microlesions. AJNR 18: 965-72, 1997

Craniopharyngioma (CP)

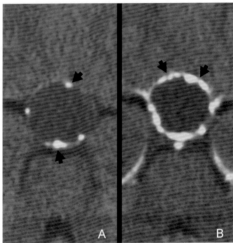

3-year-old male. NECT scan (A) shows a cystic suprasellar mass with a partially calcified wall (arrows). Cyst fluid is slightly hyperdense to CSF. (B) CECT scan shows strong rim enhancement (arrows). Craniopharyngioma.

Key Facts
- Most common suprasellar mass in children
- Two types, adamantinomatous and papillary
- Bimodal age distribution (larger peak in childhood)

Imaging Findings
General Features
- Solid tumor with variable cystic component
- Best diagnostic sign= Ca++ cystic suprasellar mass in a child

CT Findings
- NECT: 90% cystic, 90% Ca++
- CECT: 90% enhance (solid nodule + rim or capsule)

MR Findings
- Variable signal intensity, often mixed
  - Iso-, hyperintense on T1WI
  - Hyper- +/- hypointense Ca++ on T2WI
  - Cyst doesn't suppress with FLAIR
- May see hyperintensity extend posteriorly along optic radiations (compression, not tumor spread)

Other Modality Findings
- DSA: Avascular with ICAs, AChAs displaced laterally, BA displaced posteriorly, penetrating branches stretched around mass

Imaging Recommendations
- MR with contrast

Differential Diagnosis
Rathke Cleft Cyst (RCC)
- Noncalcified, usually doesn't enhance
- Small RCC may be indistinguishable from intrasellar CP

Craniopharyngioma (CP)

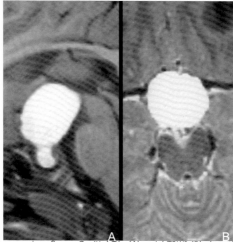

Same case as previous figure. Sagittal T1- (A), axial T2WI (B) show the mass has intra, suprasellar components and is hyperintense on both sequences.

<u>Xanthogranuloma</u>
- Preferential occurrence in adolescents, young adults
- Smaller, predominantly intrasellar, mass

<u>Thrombosed Aneurysm</u>
- Older patients
- Contains blood products
- Look for residual patent lumen

Pathology

<u>General</u>
- General Path Comments
  - 70% suprasellar mass + smaller intrasellar component
  - Only 5% purely intrasellar
  - May extend behind clivus, into multiple cranial fossae
  - Rare: CP entirely within third ventricle
- Genetics
  - No known genetic susceptibility
- Embryology
  - Anterior wall of Rathke pouch develops into adenohypophysis
  - Remaining stomodeum develops into non-keratinized squamous epithelium (gives rise to oral mucosa, teeth)
  - Rathke pouch fails to develop normally
    - May differentiate into tooth primordia (adamantinomatous CP)
    - May differentiate into oral mucosa (squamous CP)
- Etiology-Pathogenesis-Pathophysiology
  - Maldifferentiation of Rathke pouch epithelium
- Epidemiology
  - Bimodal age distribution
    - Most common 5-15ys
    - > 50 years (papillary CPs occur almost exclusively in adults)
  - M = F

Craniopharyngioma (CP)

Gross Pathologic or Surgical Features
- Solid tumor with variable cyst(s)
- Adamantinomatous cysts often contain thick "machine oil-like" brownish yellow fluid

Microscopic Features
- Adamantinomatous
  o Multistratified squamous epithelium with nuclear palisading
  o Nodules of "wet" keratin
  o Dystrophic Ca++ common
- Papillary
  o Sheets of squamous epithelium form pseudopapillae
  o Villous fibrovascular stroma

Staging or Grading Criteria
- WHO grade I

Clinical Issues

Presentation
- Visual disturbances
  o Bitemporal hemianopsia
- Endocrine disturbances
  o GH deficiency
  o Diabetes insipidus
- Large tumors may cause hydrocephalus, headaches

Natural History
- Slowly growing benign neoplasm

Treatment & Prognosis
- Surgical resection
- 10 year survival between 60%-95%

Selected References
1. Janzer RC et al: Craniopharyngioma. In Kleihues P, Cavenee WK (eds), Tumours of the Nervous System, IARC Press, 244-6, 2000
2. Hayward R: The present and future management of childhood craniopharyngioma. Childs Nerv Syst 15: 764-9, 1999
3. Harwood-Nash DC: Neuroimaging of childhood craniopharyngioma. Pediatr Neurosurg 21 (suppl 1): 2-10, 1994

Metastatic Disease

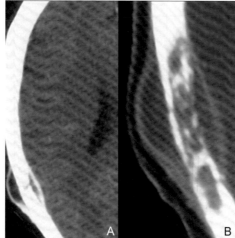

CECT scan with soft tissue (A) and magnified bone algorithm (B) show a lytic destructive calvarial mass that displaces the scalp and dura. Breast metastasis.

Key Facts
- Account for up to 50% of all brain tumors
- Found in 25% of patients with systemic cancer at autopsy

Imaging Findings
General Features
- Best diagnostic signs
  - Discrete parenchymal mass(es) at gray-white interface
  - "En plaque" or focal nodular dural mass +/- skull lesion
- Other manifestations
  - Diffuse leptomeningeal spread ("carcinomatous meningitis")
  - Pineal, pituitary, choroid plexus mass
  - Limbic encephalitis
    - Paraneoplastic syndrome (remote effect of cancer)
    - Resembles herpes encephalitis (subacute clinical presentation)

CT Findings
- Parenchyma
  - Iso- or hypodense mass at gray-white interface
  - Peritumoral edema, +/- hemorrhage
  - Intense, punctate, nodular or ring enhancement
- Dura
  - Isodense focal mass > diffuse pachymeningiopathy
  - Bone windows detect adjacent skull involvement

MR Findings
- Iso/hypo- on T1-, hyperintense on T2WI, FLAIR (melanotic melanoma, hemorrhagic lesions may be hyperintense on T1WI)
- Strong, uniform, punctate, solid or ring enhancement

Imaging Recommendations
- Contrast-enhanced MRI >> CECT
- Double or triple-contrast dose increases sensitivity but ? value on routine basis

Metastatic Disease

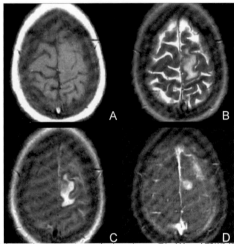

Patient with known breast carcinoma had a seizure. T1- (A) and T2WI (B), FLAIR (C) scans show a small mass at the GW junction with surrounding edema. (D) The lesion enhances strongly. Solitary metastasis.

Differential Diagnosis
Ring-Enhancing Mass (Single or Multiple)
- Abscess (usually show increased signal on DWI, reduced ADC)
- Primary neoplasm (e.g., GBM)
- Other: Demyelinating disease, resolving hematoma, etc.

Multifocal White Matter Lesions
- If it doesn't enhance, it probably isn't metastatic disease

Pathology
General
- General Path Comments
  - Location
    - 80% found at hemisphere arterial border zones
    - 15% cerebellum, 3% basal ganglia
  - Number
    - 50% have solitary metastasis
    - 20% two metastases, 30% three or more
- Genetics
  - Metastasis formation is complex event
    - Inactivation of tumor suppressor genes
    - Activation of proto-oncogenes
  - Organ-specific metastasis formation
    - Specific receptors mediate attachment, infiltration of circulating tumor cells into CNS
    - Chromosome 17q (RHO gene family), 8q (c-myc) gains
    - Overexpression, amplification of EGFR gene
  - Some tumor-specific patterns of disease spread
    - ER+/PR+ breast cancers osseous > brain metastases
    - ER-/PR- tumors brain > osseous metastases

Metastatic Disease

- Etiology-Pathogenesis
  - o Hematogenous spread (extracranial primary neoplasm)
    - Lung, breast, melanoma
    - 10% unknown primary
  - o Geographic extension
    - Tumor extension to dura from calvarium
    - Directly through skull base or via foramina, fissures (e.g., nasopharyngeal SCCA)
    - Perineural or perivascular
  - o "Brain to brain" spread from primary CNS neoplasm (e.g., GBM)
- Epidemiology
  - o Increasing prevalence in last 3 decades
  - o Now account for up to 50% of all brain tumors
  - o Seen in 25% of cancer patients at autopsy

Gross Pathologic or Surgical Features
- Round/confluent, relatively discrete tan or grayish-white mass
- Metastases usually displace rather than infiltrate tissue

Microscopic Features
- Usually similar to primary neoplasm
- Necrosis, neovascularity common

Clinical Issues

Presentation
- Seizure, focal neurologic deficit

Natural History
- Progressive enlargement
- Marked mitoses; labelling index may be greater than primary

Treatment & Prognosis
- Varies with number of metastases, location
- Mean survival with whole brain XRT = 3-6 months
- Resection of solitary metastasis may improve survival

Selected References
1. Kleinschmidt-DeMasters BK: Dural metastases: A retrospective surgical and autopsy series. Arch Pathol Lab Med 125: 880-7, 2001
2. Nelson JS et al: Metastatic tumours of the CNS in Kleihues P, Cavanee WK (eds), Tumours of the Nervous System, 250-3, IARC Press, 2000
3. Maki DD et al: Patterns of disease spread in metastatic breast carcinoma: Influence of estrogen and progesterone receptor status. AJNR 21: 1064-6, 2000

Paraneoplastic Syndromes (PSs)

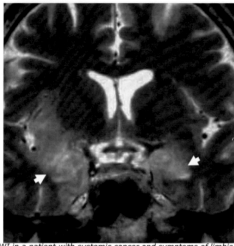

Coronal T2WI in a patient with systemic cancer and symptoms of limbic encephalitis shows bilateral but asymmetric high signal (white arrows) in both temporal lobes.

Key Facts
- PSs = remote neurological effect(s) of cancer
- Spectrum of neurologic manifestations
- Associated with extra-CNS tumors (most common = small cell lung carcinomas)
- Occurs in < 1% of patients with systemic cancer
- Majority have no known primary neoplasm at initial presentation
- Limbic encephalitis is most common clinical PS

Imaging Findings
General Features (limbic encephalitis)
- Best diagnostic sign = looks like herpes encephalitis but different clinical course (subacute/chronic >> acute)
CT Findings
- NECT
  - Initial CT scan normal in >95%
  - Rare: Low density within mesial temporal lobes
- CECT: Usually no visible enhancement
MR Findings
- Initial study normal in 20-40%
- T2/FLAIR hyperintensity
  - 75% bilateral
  - Mesial temporal lobes (hippocampus, amygdala), insula
  - Cingulate gyrus
  - Subfrontal cortex/inferior frontal WM
- Mass effect minimal/absent
- Patchy enhancement common
- No hemorrhage!
Other Modality Findings
- None reported

Paraneoplastic Syndromes (PSs)

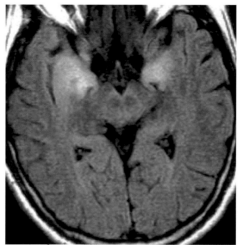

Same case as previous figure. Axial FLAIR sequence demonstrates high signal intensity in both hippocampi. The lesions enhanced minimally (not shown). Paraneoplastic syndrome.

<u>Imaging Recommendations</u>
- Repeat MR if initial scan normal + high clinical suspicion

Differential Diagnosis
<u>Herpes Encephalitis</u>
- Rapid onset, febrile illness
- HSV titers (CSF, serum) negative
- Mass effect common
- Late acute/subacute may hemorrhage
- Restricted diffusion reported
- May be indistinguishable from limbic encephalitis

<u>Neoplasm</u>
- Low grade glioma
  - Unilateral
  - No enhancement
- Gliomatosis cerebri
  - Diffuse process (no predilection for limbic system)
  - Enlarges affected area
- Metastases (multifocal enhancing lesions)

<u>Seizures/Status Epilepticus</u>
- Abnormal T2/FLAIR mesial temporal lobes, cortical enhancement
- Clinical information

Pathology
<u>General</u>
- General Path Comments
  - PSs divided into disorders of
    - CNS: Paraneoplastic cerebellar degeneration, opsoclonus/ myoclonus, retinopathy
    - Peripheral NS: Sensory-motor neuropathy, autonomic neuropathy

Paraneoplastic Syndromes (PSs)

- Both CNS/PNS: Encephalomyelitis (limbic encephalitis, brain stem encephalitis, myelitis, motor neuron disease);
- Neuromuscular junction: Lambert-Eaton myasthenic syndrome
  - o Limbic encephalitis is most common PS
    - Hippocampus, cingulate gyrus, pyriform cortex, frontal orbital surface of temporal lobe, insula, amygdala
- Etiology-Pathogenesis-Pathophysiology
  - o Immune-mediated
  - o 60% of patients have circulating serum autoantibodies
    - Anti-Hu (lung cancer), limbic encephalitis
    - Anti-Ta (testicular germ-cell tumors), limbic encephalitis
    - Anti-Yo (breast & ovarian Ca), cerebellar degeneration
- Epidemiology
  - o <1% of patients with systemic cancers develop PS

Gross Pathologic, Surgical Features
- Ill-defined softening, discoloration of GM

Microscopic Features
- Neuronal loss, reactive gliosis, perivascular infiltration of lymphocytes, microglial nodules
- **No** neoplasm! **No** viral inclusions!

Clinical Issues

Presentation
- Subacute >> acute
  - o Afebrile
  - o Cognitive dysfunction, severe memory loss, psychological features (anxiety, depression, hallucinations), seizures
- 90% have + CSF (pleocytosis, elevated protein, oligoclonal bands)
- Up to 60% have no known primary tumor at presentation; many have no tumor found at workup
- Primary neoplasm
  - o Most common = lung (small cell)
  - o Other = GI, GU (ovary>renal>uterus), Hodgkin's lymphoma, breast, testicular, thymus, neuroblastoma (pediatric)

Natural History
- Relates to primary neoplasm
- Relates to type of PS
  - o Slow long-term cognitive decline (limbic encephalitis)
  - o Progressive ataxia, weakness (cerebellar, spinal cord degeneration)

Treatment & Prognosis
- Treatment of primary malignancy may improve neurologic symptoms (25% - 45%)

Selected References
1. Gultekin SH et al: Paraneoplastic limbic encephalitis: neurological symptoms, immunological findings and tumour association in 50 patients. Brain 123: 1481-94, 2000
2. Scaravilli F et al: The Neuropathology of Paraneoplastic Syndromes. Brain Pathol 9:251-60, 1999
3. Kodama T et al: Magnetic resonance imaging of limbic encephalitis. Neuroradiology 33:520-3, 1991

CYSTS

Arachnoid Cyst

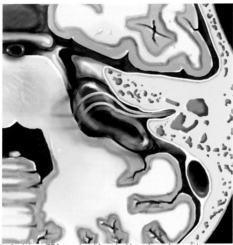

Axial graphic depicts a CPA arachnoid cyst. Vessels and cranial nerves are displaced around the cyst.

Key Facts
- Arachnoid layers contains CSF
- Middle cranial fossa = most common site

Imaging Findings
General Features
- Best diagnostic sign = sharply demarcated round/ovoid CSF cyst
- Displays features of extra-axial mass
  - Displaces cortex
  - "Buckles" gray-white interface
- If in middle fossa, temporal lobe may appear hypoplastic
CT Findings
- NECT
  - Usually CSF density
    - Intracyst hemorrhage (rare)
    - Subdural hematoma (increased prevalence)
  - May expand, remodel bone
  - CT cisternography demonstrates presence/absence of communication with subarachnoid space
- CECT: Doesn't enhance
MR Findings
- Signal parallels CSF on all sequences
- Suppresses completely with FLAIR
Other Modality Findings
- DWI: No restriction
Imaging Recommendations
- MR + DWI

Arachnoid Cyst

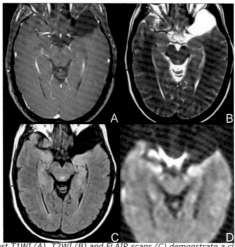

Post-contrast T1WI (A), T2WI (B) and FLAIR scans (C) demonstrate a classic middle fossa arachnoid cyst. The nonenhancing cyst follows CSF on all sequences. (D) DWI shows no restriction.

Differential Diagnosis

Epidermoid Cyst
- Scalloped margins
- Insinuating growth pattern
  - Creeps along, into CSF cisterns
  - Surrounds, engulfs vessels and nerves
- Doesn't suppress on FLAIR
- Shows restricted diffusion (bright) on DWI

Other Congenital/Inflammatory Cyst
- Cysticercosis
  - Scolex
  - Often appears conglomerate, multiloculated
- Neurenteric cyst
  - Rare
  - Often proteinaceous fluid

Cystic Neoplasm (e.g., Cystic Schwannoma)
- Some peripheral enhancement
- CN VIII schwannoma often enlarges IAC

Pathology

General
- General Path Comments
  - Fluid-containing cyst with translucent membrane
- Embryology
  - Old = "splitting" or diverticulum of developing arachnoid
  - New (middle fossa ACs)
    - Frontal, temporal embryonic meninges (endomeninx) fail to merge as sylvian fissure forms
    - Remain separate, forming "duplicated" arachnoid

Arachnoid Cyst

- Etiology-Pathogenesis
  - Possible mechanisms
    - Active fluid secretion by cyst wall
    - Slow distention by CSF pulsations
    - CSF accumulates by one-way (ball-valve) flow
  - Rare: ACs may form as shunt complication
- Epidemiology
  - 1% of intracranial masses
  - ACs found at any age; 75% in children
  - M:F = 3-5:1

Gross Pathologic or Surgical Features
- Arachnoid bulges around CSF-like cyst
  - 50% middle cranial fossa
  - 10% suprasellar (SSAC)
    - Noncommunicating = cyst of the membrane of Liliequist
    - Communicating = cystic dilation of interpeduncular cistern
  - 5%-10% CPA
  - Other: Quadrigeminal cistern, convexity
- ACs displace but don't engulf vessels, CNs

Microscopic Features
- Wall consists of flattened but normal arachnoid cells
- No inflammation, neoplastic change

Clinical Issues

Presentation
- Often asymptomatic, found incidentally
- Headache, dizziness, SNHL, hemifacial spasm/tic
- SSACs may cause obstructive hydrocephalus

Natural History
- May (but usually don't) slowly enlarge

Treatment & Prognosis
- Treatment: Often none
- Resection/fenestration (may be endoscopic), shunt if symptomatic

Selected References
1. Miyajima M et al: Possible origin of suprasellar arachnoid cysts: neuroimaging and neurosurgical observations in nine cases. J Neurosurg 93: 62-7, 2000
2. Wester K: Peculariaties of intracranial arachnoid cysts: Location, sidedness, and sex distribution in 126 consecutive patients. Neurosurg 45: 775-9, 1999
3. Oberbauer RW et al: Arachnoid cysts in children: a European cooperative study. Childs Nerv Syst 8: 281-6, 1992

Colloid Cyst

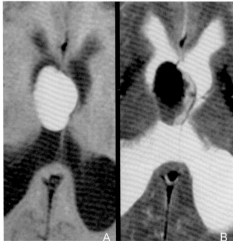

66-year old male with severe headaches. Large foramen of Monro mass is hyperintense on T1- (A) and mixed iso/hypointense on T2WI (B). Note obstructive hydrocephalus. Colloid cyst.

Key Facts
- Benign mass in anterior 3rd ventricle/foramen of Monro
- Location, imaging features characteristic
- May cause acute hydrocephalus, sudden death

Imaging Findings
General Features
- Well-demarcated round/ovoid gelatinous cyst
- Mean size = 15mm
- Best diagnostic sign = hyperdense spherical mass (NECT)
  - Located in anterior third ventricle at foramen of Monro
  - Splays posterior part of frontal horns around itself

CT Findings
- NECT
  - 2/3 hyperdense (Ca++ rare)
  - 1/3 iso/hypodense
  - +/- Hydrocephalus
- CECT
  - Usually doesn't enhance
  - Rare = rim enhancement

MR Findings
- Signal intensity varies with cyst content
  - Iso/hyperintense on T1WI
  - Variable (hypo/hyperintense) on T2WI
    - May have central marked hypointensity ("black hole" effect)
    - Rare = fluid-fluid level
- May show peripheral enhancement
- May have associated ventriculomegaly

Colloid Cyst

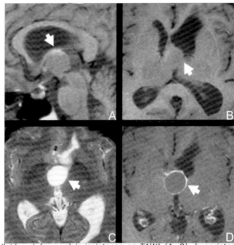

Atypical colloid cyst (arrows) is isointense on T1WI (A, B), hyperintense on T2WI (C), and shows rim enhancement (D).

Differential Diagnosis

<u>Neurocysticercosis</u>
- Multiple lesions within parenchyma and cisterns
- Associated ependymitis or basilar meningitis
- Isodense to CSF on CT
- Look for scolex

<u>CSF Flow Artifact (MR "Pseudocyst")</u>
- Multiplanar technique confirms artifact
- Look for phase artifact

<u>Vertebrobasilar Dolichoectasia/Aneurysm</u>
- Extreme VBD can cause foramen of Monro mass
- Look for "flow void," phase artifact

<u>Neoplasm</u>
- Subependymoma
  - Frontal horn of lateral ventricle
  - Attached to septum pellucidum
  - Patchy/solid enhancement
- Choroid plexus papilloma
  - Rare in 3rd ventricle
  - Tumor of early childhood

Pathology

<u>General</u>
- General Path Comments
  - Location
    - Typically anterior 3rd ventricle at foramen of Monro
    - Attached to 3rd ventricular roof and choroid plexus
    - Rarely involves septum pellucidum or fornices
    - Uncommon sites: Meninges, 4th ventricle

Colloid Cyst

- Etiology-Pathogenesis
  - From embryonic endoderm, **not** neuroectoderm!
- Epidemiology
  - 0.5% to 1.0% primary brain tumors
  - 15% to 20% intraventricular masses

Gross Pathologic or Surgical Features
- Smooth, spherical, well-delineated cystic lesion 3 mm – 4 cm
- Collagenous capsule with underlying epithelium
- Gelatinous center, variable viscosity (mucinous or desiccated)
- +/- Blood products, cholesterol, various ions (Ca++, etc.)

Microscopic Features
- Thin outer fibrous capsule
- Inner lining = single layer of flat cuboidal/low columnar epithelium
- Cyst contents = PAS+ gelatinous colloid material

Clinical Issues
Presentation
- 40%-50% asymptomatic
- 50%-60% symptomatic
  - Present between 20-50yr (rare in children)
  - Headache = common presenting symptom
  - Less common = nausea, vomiting, memory loss, altered personality, gait disturbance, visual changes
- Acute foramen of Monro obstruction may lead to rapid onset hydrocephalus, herniation, death

Natural History
- >90% don't change size
- May enlarge (e.g., hemorrhage), occasionally shrink

Treatment & Prognosis
- Most common treatment = surgical resection
- Options include stereotactic aspiration, endoscopic resection, ventricular shunting, observation (rare)
- Imaging features may predict difficulty with percutaneous therapy
  - Hyperdensity on CT/hypointensity on T2WI suggest high viscosity, possibly difficult aspiration

Selected References
1. Jeffree RL et al: Colloid cyst of the third ventricle: a clinical review of 39 cases. J Clinical Neurosci 8: 328-31, 2001
2. Pollack BE et al: A theory of the natural history of colloid cysts of the third ventricle. Neurosurgery 46:1077-83, 2000
3. Kirsch CFE et al: Colloid cysts. IJNR 3: 460-9, 1997

Enlarged Perivascular Spaces

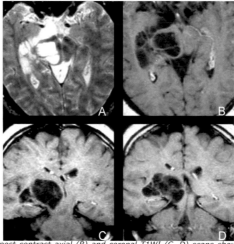

T2WI (A), post-contrast axial (B) and coronal T1WI (C, D) scans show expanding ("tumefactive") PVSs causing midbrain mass effect.

Key Facts
- Prominent perivascular (Virchow-Robin) spaces (PVSs) are seen at all ages, in many locations
- PVSs are lined by pia, contain interstitial fluid (ISF)
- PVSs do not communicate directly with subarachnoid space
- Clusters of enlarged PVSs may cause mass effect, hydrocephalus

Imaging Findings
General Features
- Best diagnostic sign = fluid-filled spaces that surround, accompany penetrating arteries
- Basal ganglia, midbrain, white matter most common sites
- Others
  - Thalami
  - Dentate nuclei
  - Subinsular cortex, extreme capsule

CT Findings
- Round/ovoid/linear/punctate
- Attenuation like CSF
- Don't enhance

MR Findings
- Single or multiple cyst-like spaces
  - Well-delineated, sharply marginated
  - Signal virtually identical to CSF on T1-, T2WI
  - Complete suppression on FLAIR
  - Adjacent parenchyma usually normal
    - No edema, enhancement
    - Minimal/mild surrounding gliosis in < 25%
- +/- Visualization of penetrating arteries with contrast
- PVSs usually 5 mm or less
  - Occasionally expand, attain large size

Enlarged Perivascular Spaces

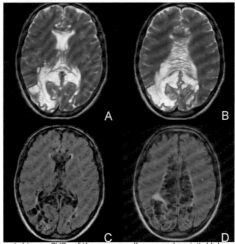

Very prominent, bizarre PVSs of the corpus callosum and occipital lobes are shown in these axial T2WI (A, B) and FLAIR (C, D) scans (courtesy L. Valanne).

- o   May cause focal mass effect, hydrocephalus
- o   Widespread dilatation of PVSs may look very bizarre

Other Modality Findings
- •   DWI: No restricted diffusion

Imaging Recommendations
- •   Routine MR + FLAIR
- •   Contrast optional

Differential Diagnosis

Lacunar Infarcts
- •   Older patients
- •   Common in basal ganglia, white matter
- •   Adjacent parenchymal hyperintensity

Cystic Neoplasm
- •   Usually in pons, cerebellum, hypothalamus
- •   Signal not quite like CSF
- •   Parenchymal signal abnormalities common
- •   May enhance

Inflammatory Cysts
- •   Neurocysticercosis cysts often have scolex
- •   Surrounding edema
- •   Usually enhance

Pathology

General
- •   General Path Comments
  - o   Enlarged cystic-appearing spaces
- •   Genetics
  - o   Usually normal unless PVSs expanded by undegraded mucopolysaccharides (Hurler, Hunter disease)
  - o   PVSs expand in some congenital muscular dystrophies

Enlarged Perivascular Spaces

- Etiology-Pathogenesis
  - Theory = ISF accumulates between penetrating vessel, pia
- Epidemiology
  - Prominent PVSs occur in all locations, at all ages
  - Present in 25%-30% of children (benign normal variant)

Gross Pathologic or Surgical Features
- Smoothly demarcated, fluid-filled cyst(s)

Microscopic Features
- Single or double layer of invaginated pia
- Pia becomes fenestrated, disappears at capillary level
- PVSs usually very small in cortex, often enlarge in subcortical white matter

Clinical Issues

Presentation
- Usually normal, discovered incidentally at imaging/autopsy
- Nonspecific symptoms (e.g., headache)

Natural History
- Usually remain stable in size
- Occasionally continue to expand

Treatment & Prognosis
- "Leave me alone" lesion that should not be mistaken for serious disease
- Shunt ventricles if midbrain lesions cause obstructive hydrocephalus

Selected References
1. Song CJ et al: MR imaging and histologic features of subinsular bright spots on T2-weighted MR images: Virchow-Robin spaces of the extreme capsule and insular cortex. Radiol 214: 671-7, 2000
2. Masalchi M et al: Expanding lacunae causing triventricular hydrocephalus. J Neurosurg 91: 669-74, 1999
3. Adachi M et al: Dilated Virchow-Robin spaces: MRI pathological study. Neuroradiol 40: 27-31, 1998

Epidermoid Cyst

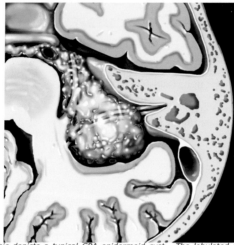

Axial graphic depicts a typical CPA epidermoid cyst. The lobulated pearly mass infiltrates the subarachnoid space, encasing both cranial nerves and blood vessels.

Key Facts
- 1% of all intracranial tumors
- Nonneoplastic inclusion cyst
- Third most common CPA/IAC mass
- Usually resembles CSF on imaging studies

Imaging Findings
General Features
- Lobulated, irregular, "cauliflower-like" pearly mass
- Best diagnostic sign= CSF-like mass insinuates into cisterns, encases nerves/vessels
CT Findings
- NECT
  - > 95% hypodense (resemble CSF)
  - 10%-25% Ca++
  - Rare variant = "dense" epidermoid
- CECT: Usually no enhancement (margin of cyst may show minimal)
MR Findings
- Signal intensity often =/ slightly > CSF on all standard sequences
- Doesn't null on FLAIR
Other Imaging Findings
- DWI: Restricted diffusion (high signal)

Differential Diagnosis
Arachnoid Cyst
- Suppresses on FLAIR
- No restricted diffusion
Inflammatory Cyst (e.g., Cysticercosis)
- Often enhances
- Density/signal intensity usually not precisely like CSF
- Edema, gliosis common

Epidermoid Cyst

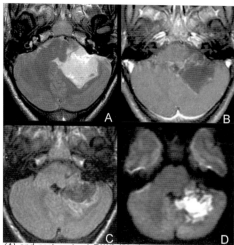

Axial T2WI (A) and post-contrast T1WI (B) show a cauliflower-shaped CPA mass with CSF-like signal intensity. (C) The lesion doesn't suppress on FLAIR. (D) DWI shows striking restricted diffusion. Epidermoid cyst.

Cystic Neoplasm
- Attenuation/signal intensity not = CSF
- Often enhances

Dermoid Cyst
- Usually at or near midline
- Resembles fat, not CSF (contains dermal appendages)

Pathology
General
- General Path Comments
  - Most occur off-midline
  - Posterior fossa = most common site
    - CPA 75%
    - Fourth ventricle 20%
    - 5% other (suprasellar, sylvian fissure)
  - Miscellaneous= skull (intradiploic), spine
- Genetics
  - Sporadic
- Embryology
  - Arise from ectodermal inclusions during neural tube closure
  - Congenital intradural CPA epidermoids derived from cells of first branchial groove
- Epidemiology
  - 1% of all intracranial neoplasms and tumorlike masses

Gross Pathologic or Surgical Features
- Pearly white ("beautiful tumor")
- Lobulated excrescences
- Insinuating growth pattern (extends through cisterns, surrounds and encases vessels/nerves)

Epidermoid Cyst

Microscopic Features
- Cyst wall = simple stratified cuboidal squamous epithelium
- Cyst contents = solid crystalline cholesterol, keratinaceous debris

Clinical Issues
Presentation
- May remain clinically silent for many years
- Presents at 20-60y (peak at 40y)
- Symptoms depend on location, growth pattern
  - Headache
  - CNs V, VII, VIII neuropathy common

Natural History
- Grows slowly

Treatment & Prognosis
- Microsurgical resection
- Recurrence common if incompletely removed

Selected References
1. Chen S et al: Quantitative MR evaluation of intracranial epidermoid tumors by fast FLAIR imaging and echo-planar DWI. AJNR 22: 1089-96, 2001
2. Kallmes DF et al: Typical and atypical MR imaging features of intracranial epidermoid tumors. AJR 169: 883-7, 1997
3. Smirniotopoulos JG et al: Teratomas, dermoids, and epidermoids of the head and neck. RadioGraphics 15: 1437-55, 1995

Dermoid Cyst

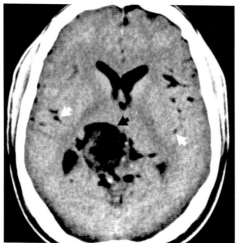

NECT scan shows hypodense mass (black arrow) with multiple low-density droplets in the subarachnoid spaces (white arrows).

Key Facts
- Intracranial dermoids are congenital inclusion cysts
- Secretions, desquamated epithelial debris cause slow expansion
- May rupture, causing significant morbidity/mortality

Imaging Findings
General Features
- Well-circumscribed unilocular cyst
- Usually midline
  - Most often in sellar/parasellar region
  - Scalp mass (2/3rds near anterior fontanelle)
  - Other sites = spine, orbit
- Best diagnostic sign = fat + droplets in cisterns, sulci, ventricles
CT Findings
- NECT
  - Round/lobulated cystic mass
  - Fat density (rare = "dense" dermoid)
  - 20% Ca++
  - With rupture, droplets of fat disseminate in cisterns, may cause fat-fluid level within ventricles
  - Skull/scalp dermoid expands diploe
  - Frontonasal: Bifid crista galli, large foramen cecum + sinus tract
- CECT: Generally no enhancement
MR Findings
- T1WI: Cyst, "rupture droplets" very hyperintense
  - Fat suppression sequence confirms
  - Fat-fluid level in cyst, ventricles common
- T2WI: Often heterogeneous
  - Chemical shift artifact in frequency encoding direction

Dermoid Cyst

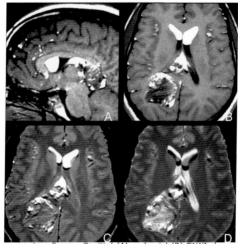

Same case as previous figure. Sagittal (A) and axial (B) T1WI show mixed signal mass with multiple hyperintense foci in the ventricles and subarachnoid spaces. PD-(C) and T2WI (D) show prominent chemical shift artifact. Ruptured dermoid (courtesy T. Swallow).

Imaging Recommendations
- Use fat-suppression sequence to confirm diagnosis
- 3D chemical shift-selective sequence useful to detect tiny droplets

Differential Diagnosis
Teratoma
- Location similar
- Has endodermal, mesenchymal elements
- Often multicystic/multiloculated
Craniopharyngioma
- Suprasellar
- Enhances
Epidermoid
- Most epidermoid cysts resemble CSF, not fat

Pathology
General
- General Path Comments
  - Can occur as scalp, skull, or intradural extra-axial mass
- Genetics
  - Sporadic, not familial
- Embryology (two theories)
  - Sequestration of surface ectoderm at lines of epithelial fusion/ along the course of normal embryonic invaginations
  - Inclusion of cutaneous ectoderm at time of neural tube closure

Dermoid Cyst

- Etiology-Pathogenesis
  - Three classifications of dermoid inclusions, based on pathogenesis
    - Congenital cystic teratoma (true neoplasm derived from all three embryonic germ layers)
    - Congenital dermoid inclusion cyst (nonneoplastic epithelial-lined inclusion cyst)
    - Acquired implantation cyst (trauma, surgery, LP)
  - 50% of congenital dermoids associated with other anomalies
    - Anterior neuropore defects (any mixture of dermoid, epidermoid, dural sinus tract)
  - Dermoid, epidermoid inclusion cysts are most common skull, scalp lesions in children
- Epidemiology
  - Rare; account for < 0.5% of primary intracranial tumors
  - Majority supratentorial, midline or near midline

Gross Pathologic or Surgical Features
- Unilocular cyst with thick wall of connective tissue
- Contents = mixture of greasy lipid, cholesterol debris
- Often contains hair

Microscopic Features
- Outer wall of fibrous connective tissue
- Lining of keratinized squamous epithelium, dermal appendages (sebaceous glands, sweat glands, hair follicles)
- Desquamated keratin, cellular debris
- Teeth with dental enamel may be present

Clinical Issues

Presentation
- Uncomplicated dermoid: Seizure, HA most common symptoms
- Cyst rupture causes chemical ("Mollaret's") meningitis

Natural History
- Benign, slow growing
- Larger lesions associated with higher rupture rate
- Rupture may cause seizure, coma, vasospasm, death
- Dermoid + dermal sinus may cause infection, hydrocephalus

Treatment & Prognosis
- Complete microsurgical excision
- Residual capsule leads to recurrence

Selected References
1. Calabro F et al: Rupture of spinal dermoid tumors with spread of fatty droplets in the CSF pathways. Neuroradiol 42: 572-9, 2000
2. Dagher AP et al: Intracranial cysts with and without rupture. IJNR 1: 134-44, 1995
3. Smirniotopoulos JG et al: Teratomas, dermoids, and epidermoids of the head and neck. RadioGraphics 15: 1437-55, 1995

Choroid Plexus Cysts

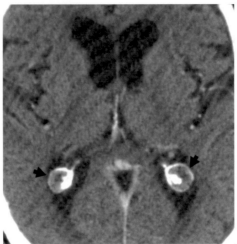

CECT scan in an asymptomatic 68-yea- old male shows bilateral, calcified, rim-enhancing cysts (arrows) in the choroid plexus glomi. Xanthogranulomas.

Key Facts
- Common incidental finding on imaging studies in older patients
- CSF-appearing cysts in choroid plexus glomi

Imaging Findings
General Features
- Cystic or nodular/partially cystic mass(es)
- Usually small (2-8mm), often multiple
- Best diagnostic sign: Older patient with CSF-like cysts in trigones

CT Findings
- NECT: Density similar to CSF
- CECT: Varies from none to rim or solid enhancement

MR Findings
- Hypo- on T1-, hyperintense on PD/T2WI (compared to brain)
- 2/3rd iso-, 1/3rd hypointense on FLAIR
- May enhance with contrast (solid, ring, nodular)

Other Modality Findings
- DWI: 65% show restricted diffusion (high signal)
- Prenatal U/S: Small fetal choroid plexus cysts common, normal

Imaging Recommendations
- MR without/with contrast, FLAIR

Differential Diagnosis
Benign Cyst
- Inflammatory (cysticercosis)
- Ependymal
  - Usually juxta- rather than intraventricular
  - Don't enhance
  - Immunoreactivity for GFAP, S-100
- Epidermoid (usually in 4th, rare in lateral ventricle)

Choroid Plexus Cysts

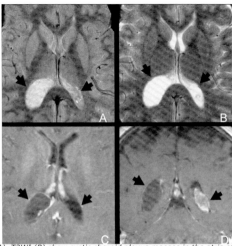

Axial PD- (A), T2WI (B) show cystic choroid plexus masses in the atria of both lateral ventricles (arrows). Post-contrast axial (C), coronal (D) T1WI show right lateral ventricular mass is hyperintense to CSF; the left atrial mass enhances. Both are xanthogranulomas (courtesy R.Sherry).

<u>Villous Hyperplasia</u>
* Often overproduces CSF

<u>Neoplasm</u>
* Choroid plexus papilloma (children <10y)
* Meningioma (usually solid)
* Metastasis
* Cystic astrocytoma (rare in older patients)

Pathology

<u>General</u>
* General Path Comments
  * Solitary or multiple fluid-filled cysts
    * Atria of lateral ventricles most common site
    * Less common: 3rd ventricle
  * Attached to or within choroid plexus
* Genetics
  * Large fetal choroid plexus cysts associated with trisomy 18
* Etiology-Pathogenesis
  * Lipid from desquamating, degenerating choroid epithelium accumulates
  * Lipid provokes xanthomatous response
* Epidemiology
  * Most common type of neuroepithelial cyst
    * 1% prevalence in fetuses
    * 1.6%-7% overall prevalence in adults
  * Incidence increases with age

<u>Gross Pathologic or Surgical Features</u>
* Nodular, partly cystic yellowish gray masses in choroid plexus glomus
* Rare: Hemorrhage

Choroid Plexus Cysts

Microscopic Features
- Nests of foamy, lipid-laden histiocytes
- Foreign body giant cells
- Chronic inflammatory infiltrates (lymphocytes, plasma cells)
- Cholesterol clefts, hemosiderin, Ca++
- Immunohistochemistry: + For prealbumin, cytokeratins; GFAP
- Trapped choroid plexus epithelium

Clinical Issues
Presentation
- Discovered incidentally at autopsy/imaging
- Occasional: Headache

Natural History
- Usually remain asymptomatic, nonprogressive
- Fetal choroid plexus cysts usually regress spontaneously

Treatment & Prognosis
- Usually none
- Rare: Shunt for obstructive hydrocephalus

Selected References
1. Ishiyama H et al: Diffusion-weighted MRI of choroid plexus cysts (abstr). Neuroradiol 43: 107, 2001
2. Boockvar JA et al: Symptomatic lateral ventricular ependymal cysts: Criteria for distinguishing these rare cysts from other symptomatic cysts of the ventricles. Neurosurg 46: 1229-33, 2000
3. Kadota T et al: MR of xanthogranuloma of the choroid plexus. AJNR 17: 1595-7, 1996

Pineal Cysts

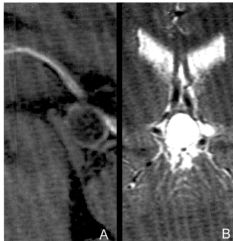

Typical cyst of the pineal gland is illustrated. Sagittal post-contrast T1WI (A) and coronal T2WI (B) show the cyst signal is similar to CSF. Enhancing rim is compressed normal pineal tissue.

Key Facts
- Pineal cysts are common incidental finding at imaging, autopsy
- Usually small, asymptomatic but may enlarge, even hemorrhage

Imaging Findings
General Features
- Round/ovoid, relatively thin-walled cyst
  - Above tectum, below ICV
  - May flatten tectum, occasionally compress aqueduct
- Best diagnostic sign: Homogeneous fluid-filled mass above, clearly distinct from tectum

CT Findings
- NECT
  - Sharply-demarcated, smooth cyst at back of 3rd ventricle
    - Fluid iso-/slightly hyperdense to CSF
    - 25% Ca++ in cyst wall
- CECT
  - Rim or nodular enhancement

MR Findings
- Variable intensity
  - 40% isointense with CSF on T1-, T2WI
  - 85%-90% hyperintense to CSF on PD (long TR/short TE)
  - May be heterogeneous, with hemorrhage/mass effect
- 60% enhance
  - Partial/complete rim, nodular
  - May fill in on delayed scans, resemble solid tumor

Imaging Recommendations
- If typical cyst found incidentally, can usually be followed on clinical basis alone (rather than imaging)

Pineal Cysts

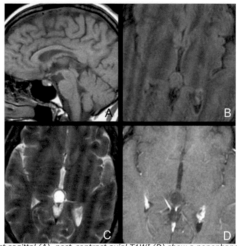

Pre-contrast sagittal (A), post-contrast axial T1WI (D) show a nonenhancing mass at the posterior third ventricle that expands the pineal gland, is slightly hyperintense to CSF on both T1-/T2WI (C), and doesn't suppress on FLAIR (B). Nonneoplastic pineal cyst.

Differential Diagnosis

Normal Pineal Gland
- Three anatomic appearances
  - Nodule (52%)
  - Crescent (26%)
  - Ring-like (22%)

Pineocytoma
- May be indistinguishable on imaging studies, require histology for definitive diagnosis
- Both pineal cyst, pineocytoma may not change on serial imaging

Pathology

General
- Embryology
  - Primitive pineal diverticulum divides into pineal recess, cavum pineal
  - Cavum pineal usually obliterated by glial fibers
  - Incomplete obliteration may leave residual cavity
- Etiology-Pathogenesis: 3 major theories
  - Enlargement of embryonic pineal cavity (see above)
  - Ischemic glial degeneration +/- hemorrhagic expansion
  - Small pre-existing cysts enlarge with hormonal influences
- Epidemiology
  - 1%-4% prevalence at imaging
  - 20%-40% microscopic cysts at autopsy
  - F: M = 3:1

Gross Pathologic or Surgical Features
- Smooth, soft, tan to yellow cyst wall
- Fluid contents vary from clear yellow (most common) to hemorrhagic
- 80% < 10 mm

Pineal Cysts

- Can be large (reported up to 4.5 cm)

Microscopic Features
- Delicate (usually incomplete) outer fibrous layer
- Middle layer of pineal parenchyma, with/without Ca++
- Inner layer of glial tissue with variable granular bodies, hemosiderin-laden macrophages

Clinical Issues

Presentation
- Vast majority clinically silent
- Large cysts (> 1 cm) may become symptomatic
  - 50% headache (aqueduct compression, hydrocephalus)
  - 10% Parinaud syndrome (tectal compression)
  - Very rare: "Pineal apoplexy" with intracystic hemorrhage, acute hydrocephalus, sudden death
- Mean age = 28 years

Natural History
- Size generally remains unchanged
- Cystic expansion of pineal in some females begins in adolescence, decreases with aging

Treatment & Prognosis
- Usually none; atypical/symptomatic lesions may require stereotactic aspiration, biopsy, resection

Selected References
1. Barboriak DP et al: Serial MR imaging of pineal cysts: Implications for natural history and follow-up. AJR 176: 737-43, 2001
2. Engel U et al: Cystic lesions of the pineal region—MRI and pathology. Neuroradiol 42: 399-402, 2000
3. Fain JS et al: Symptomatic glial cysts of the pineal gland. J Neurosurg 80: 454-60, 1994

Rathke Cleft Cyst (RCC)

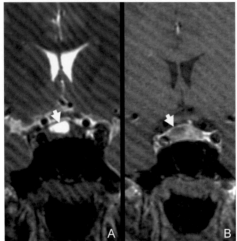

Coronal T2- (A) and post-contrast T1WI (B) show a nonenhancing intrapituitary cyst (arrows) found incidentally in this 32-year-old female with headaches. Probable Rathke cleft cyst.

Key Facts
- Common intra/suprasellar nonneoplastic cyst
- Most are asymptomatic, discovered incidentally

Imaging Findings
General Features
- Best diagnostic clue = non-enhancing, noncalcified hyperintense (T2WI) intrapituitary cyst

CT Findings
- NECT
  - Well-delineated round/lobulated intra/suprasellar mass
    - 40% intrasellar, <10mm; 60% suprasellar extension
    - 75% hypo-, 25% mixed iso/hypodense
    - 10%-15% Ca++ (curvilinear, in cyst wall)
  - Rare: Sphenoid sinusitis
- CECT
  - Doesn't enhance

MR Findings
- Can be intrapituitary (surrounded by normal gland), suprasellar, or both
- Signal varies with cyst contents (serous, mucoid)
  - 30%-40% like CSF (hypo- on T1-, hyperintense on T2WI)
  - 50%-60% hyper- on T1WI, iso-/hypointense on T2WI
  - 5%-10% mixed (may have fluid-fluid level)
- No internal enhancement (enhancing rim of compressed normal pituitary can sometimes be seen)
- 75% have small nonenhancing intracystic nodule
- Size varies (usually small; some RCCs attain large size)

Rathke Cleft Cyst (RCC)

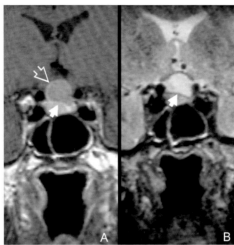

(A) Coronal contrast-enhanced MR scan shows a suprasellar mass compressing the pituitary gland. Note anterosuperior cap of enhancing pituitary (open arrow). (B) Long TR/short TE scan shows the mass is hyperintense. Rathke cleft cyst (white arrows).

Differential Diagnosis
Craniopharyngioma
- Histologic continuum between RCC, craniopharyngioma (if noncalcified, can be indistinguishable from RCC on imaging)
- Floccular Ca++ common in craniopharyngioma, rare in RCC
- 90% enhance (nodular, rim)

Cystic Pituitary Adenoma
- Ca++ rare
- Rim enhancement common

Other Nonneoplastic Cyst
- Arachnoid cyst (signal identical to CSF, no intracystic nodule)
- Miscellaneous intrasellar cyst (pars intermedia, colloid, dermoid, epidermoid cysts occur)

Pathology
General
- General Path Comments
  - One of spectrum of midline sellar/juxtasellar ectodermal cysts
- Embryology
  - Ectodermal origin (persistence of Rathke's pouch)
    - Stomodeum (primitive oral cavity) invaginates
    - Extends dorsally, forms ectodermal-lined craniopharyngeal duct
    - Meets infundibulum (outgrowth of 3rd ventricle) by 11th fetal week, gives rise to hypophysis
    - Anterior wall of pouch forms anterior lobe, pars tuberalis
    - Posterior wall forms pars intermedia
    - Lumen forms narrow cleft that normally regresses by 12th week of gestation
    - Persistence, expansion gives rise to RCC
  - Neuroepithellal or endodermal origin (less likely)

Rathke Cleft Cyst (RCC)

- Etiology-Pathogenesis
  - Arises from embryonic remnants of Rathke's pouch
- Epidemiology
  - Usually incidental, found in up to 1/3 of all autopsies

Gross Pathologic or Surgical Features
- Smoothly lobulated, well-delineated intra/suprasellar cystic mass containing clear or whitish mucoid fluid
- Location
  - Most RCCs are limited to sella
    - Between anterior, intermediate lobes
  - May become large, present as suprasellar mass

Microscopic Features
- Wall = single layer of ciliated cuboidal/columnar epithelium +/- goblet cells
- Variable cyst content
  - Clear or serous, +/- hemorrhage, hemosiderin
  - Amorphous, inspissated eosinophilic mucicarmine-positive colloid +/- cholesterol clefts
  - Firm, waxy yellow, inspissated material
- Immunohistochemical stains + for cytokeratin

Clinical Issues
Presentation
- Most are asymptomatic, incidental
- Symptomatic RCC
  - 70% pituitary dysfunction (amenorrhea/galactorrhea, DI, panhypopituitarism, hyperprolactinemia)
  - 45%-55% visual disturbances
  - 50% headache

Natural History
- Most are stable, don't change in size/signal intensity
- Some cysts may shrink/disappear spontaneously
- Iso-/hyperintense cysts on T1WI more often cause symptoms
- RCCs don't undergo neoplastic degeneration

Treatment & Prognosis
- Conservative if asymptomatic
- Aspiration/partial excision if symptomatic

Selected References
1. Byun WM et al: MR imaging findings of Rathke's cleft cysts: Significance of intracystic nodules. AJNR 21: 485-8, 2000
2. Saeki N et al: MRI findings and clinical manifestations in Rathke's cleft cyst. Acta Neurochir (Wien) 141: 1055-61, 1999
3. Kleinschmidt-DeMasters BK et al: The pathologic, surgical, and MR spectrum of Rathke cleft cysts. Surg Neurol 44: 19-27, 1995

MENINGES

Neurosarcoid (NS)

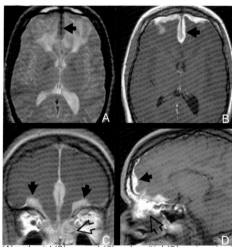

Axial T2WI (A) and axial (B), coronal (C) and sagittal (D) post-contrast T1WI show extensive bifrontal dural thickening (arrows). Note enhancing tissue in nose, ethmoid sinuses (open arrows). Sarcoid (courtesy B. Burton).

Key Facts
- Multisystem noncaseating epithelioid-cell granulomas
- Brain involved in 5% (clinical) to 25% (autopsy)
- NS can occur without evidence of systemic disease
- Protean manifestations make NS a "great mimicker"

Imaging Findings
General Features
- Best diagnostic sign = solitary or multifocal, extra-axial mass + abnormal chest x-ray
CT Findings
- Sensitivity << MRI
- May show basilar leptomeningeal enhancement
MR Findings
- Wide spectrum of brain lesions
  - Nearly half have periventricular high-signal lesions on T2WI
  - Slightly > 1/3 have multiple parenchymal lesions
  - Slightly > 1/3 have leptomeningeal enhancement (can be nodular or diffuse)
  - 10% solitary intra-axial mass
  - 5% solitary dural-based extra-axial mass
  - 5%-10% hypothalamus/pituitary stalk
  - Others: Hydrocephalus, vasculitis, lacunar infarcts (brainstem, basal ganglia), ependymal enhancement
- Can also involve spinal cord, nerve roots
Other Modality Findings
- Chest X-ray abnormal in most patients with NS
  - Hilar adenopathy +/- parenchymal involvement
  - Diffuse rcticular infiltrates
- Gallium scan (positive in majority)

Neurosarcoid (NS)

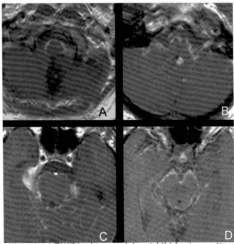

A series of post-contrast T1WI is shows nodular pial thickening coating the medulla, pons, midbrain, cerebellum, and left CNs VII and VIII. Focal dural-based masses are present along the tentorium. Sarcoid.

Differential Diagnosis

Neoplasm
- Solitary intra-axial mass mimics astrocytoma
- Dural mass (es) can mimic meningioma, metastases
- Cerebellopontine angle mass can mimic schwannoma
- Multifocal "miliary" parenchymal lesions mimic metastases

Meningitis
- Can be indistinguishable from bacterial, fungal, TB or carcinomatous meningitis

Demyelinating Disease
- Periventricular white matter lesions can mimic MS

Pathology

General
- General Path Comments
  - Focal or diffusely infiltrating granulomas involve parenchyma, leptomeninges, dura
- Etiology-Pathogenesis
  - Unknown; possibly stimulation of immune system by one or more antigens
  - No clear familial pattern, occupational/environmental exposure, infectious link
- Epidemiology
  - Onset usually in third/fourth decades (3%-5% children)
  - 10 to 20 per 100,000 in North America
  - Incidence in African-Americans 10x whites, women 2x men
  - Lung affected in > 90%
  - CNS 25% (autopsy; only 5% clinical)

Neurosarcoid (NS)

<u>Microscopic Features</u>
- Round/ovoid noncaseating granuloma composed of compact, radially arranged epithelioid cells with pale-staining nuclei
- Giant cells in arc/circle around central granular zone
- Leptomeningeal granulomas extend into perivascular (Virchow-Robin) spaces, adjacent parenchyma

Clinical Issues
<u>Presentation</u>
- Can involve any organ
- Symptoms vary with location, size of granulomas
- Skin lesions in up to 1/3
- Iritis, uveitis, polyarthritis, lymphadenopathy also common
- Neurological symptoms can occur without evidence of pulmonary or systemic sarcoidosis
  - o Cranial neuropathy (facial paralysis, diplopia/visual symptoms)
  - o Headache, fatigue, seizures
  - o Weakness, paresthesias
  - o Signs of meningeal irritation
  - o Pituitary/hypothalamic dysfunction (e.g., diabetes insipidus)
- Serum ACE levels elevated in < 50% of cases with NS
- CSF neither sensitive nor specific

<u>Natural History</u>
- Variable (some respond rapidly to steroids, others refractory)

<u>Treatment & Prognosis</u>
- Corticosteroids useful in many cases
- Immunosuppressive drugs in others

Selected References
1. Pickuth D et al: Role of radiology in the diagnosis of neurosarcoidosis. Eur Radiol 10: 941-4, 2000
2. Keesling CA et al: Clinical and imaging manifestations of pediatric sarcoidosis. Acad Radiol 5: 122-32, 1998
3. Hollander MD et al: Neuroradiology case of the day. RadioGraphics 18: 1608-11, 1998

Intracranial Hypotension

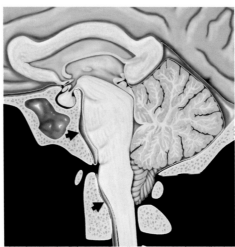

Sagittal graphic depicts the "slumping" midbrain, acquired tonsillar herniation, and engorged dura (arrows) characteristic of intracranial hypotension.

Key Facts
- Frequently misdiagnosed; imaging key to correct diagnosis
- Classic imaging triad = diffuse dural thickening, downward displacement of brain through incisura, subdural hygromas
- Lack of one classic finding does not preclude diagnosis

Imaging Findings
General Features
- Best diagnostic sign = combination of diffuse dural enhancement, "slumping midbrain"
CT Findings
- Relatively insensitive; may appear normal
MR Findings
- Smooth, diffuse dural thickening
  - Isointense with brain on T1WI, hyperintense on T2WI
  - Strong enhancement (N.B.: Absence of meningeal enhancement does not preclude diagnosis of intracranial hypotension)
- 70% have subdural hygromas (clear fluid collects within dural border cell layer); 10% have hematomas
- Downward displacement of brain
  - Sagittal
    - "Sagging" midbrain (displaced inferiorly, below level of dorsum sellae; pons may be compressed against clivus)
    - Decreased angle between peduncles, pons
    - Caudal displacement of tonsils in 25%-75%
    - Optic chiasm, hypothalamus draped over sella
  - Axial
    - Suprasellar cistern crowded/effaced
    - Elongation of midbrain ("fat midbrain")
    - Temporal lobes herniated over tentorium, into incisura

Intracranial Hypotension

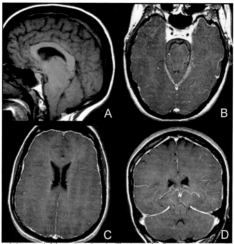

Spontaneous intracranial hypotension is illustrated. Pre-contrast sagittal T1WI (A) shows slumping midbrain, tonsillar herniation, and optic chiasm/hypothalamus draped over sella. (B-D) Post-contrast scans show dura-arachnoid thickening.

- Lateral ventricles small, often distorted by downward displacement
- Other: Dilated cervical epidural venous plexus, spinal hygromas, retrospinal fluid collections

<u>Other Modality Findings</u>
- CT myelography: May demonstrate leakage, +/- actual site
- Radioisotope cisternography (rapid washout from CSF space, rapid appearance of urinary bladder activity, +/- site of leakage)

<u>Imaging Recommendations</u>
- Search for actual leakage site only
  - If two adequate blood patches have failed
  - If post-traumatic leak is suspected

Differential Diagnosis
<u>Pachymeningiopathy</u>
- Infection, neoplasm (dura thick but midbrain in normal position)
- Dural sinus thrombosis with venous engorgement
- Idiopathic

<u>Descending Transtentorial Herniation</u>
- Diffuse cerebral edema or large focal mass
- Brain is "pushed down" rather than "sucked down"
- Dura usually normal

Pathology
<u>General</u>
- Etiology-Pathogenesis
  - Etiology = reduced CSF pressure, precipitated by
    - Surgery or trauma (including trivial fall)
    - Vigorous exercise
    - Violent coughing

- Diagnostic lumbar puncture
- Spontaneous dural tear or rupture of arachnoid diverticulum
- Severe dehydration
  - Pathophysiology = Monro-Kellie doctrine
    - CSF and intracranial blood volume vary inversely
    - In face of low CSF pressure, dural venous plexi dilate
- Epidemiology
  - M > F
  - Peak in third, fourth decades

Gross Pathologic or Surgical Features
- Usually unremarkable
- No specific leakage site identified at surgery in at least 50%

Microscopic Features
- Meningeal surface normal
- Deep surface may show marked arachnoidal and dural fibrosis with numerous dilated thin-walled vessels
- No evidence for inflammation or neoplasia

Clinical Issues

Presentation
- Severe headache (can be orthostatic, persistent, pulsatile or even associated with nuchal rigidity)
- Uncommon: CN palsy (e.g., abducens), visual disturbances
- Rare: Severe encephalopathy with disturbances of consciousness
- LP: Low CSF pressure +/- pleocytosis, increased protein

Natural History
- Most cases resolve spontaneously
- Dural thickening, enhancement disappears and midline structures return to normal position
- In rare cases, coma and death from intracranial herniation ensue

Treatment & Prognosis
- Aimed at restoring CSF volume (fluid replacement, bedrest)
- Autologous blood patch, epidural saline infusion
- Surgery if large dural tear, ruptured diverticulum or Tarlov cyst

Selected References
1. Yousry I et al: Cervical MR imaging in postural headache: MR signs and pathophysiological implications. AJNR 22: 1239-50, 2001
2. Christoforidis GA et al: Spontaneous intracranial hypotension. Neuroradiol 40: 636-43, 1998
3. Dillon WP et al: Some lessons about the diagnosis and treatment of spontaneous intracranial hypotension. AJNR 19: 1001-2, 1998

Hypertrophic Pachymeninges

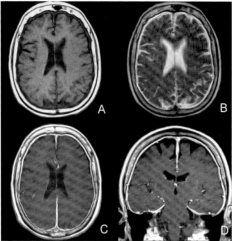

Pre-contrast axial T1- (A) and T2WI (B), post-contrast axial (C), coronal (D) T1WI show diffuse dura-arachnoid thickening. Biopsy showed dural fibrosis without tumor or inflammation. Idiopathic hypertrophic pachymeningitis.

Key Facts
- Normal dural enhancement = thin (<2 mm), discontinuous, most prominent at convexity, less intense than cavernous sinus
- Abnormal dural-arachnoid enhancement is 2 mm or greater, intense, continuous, can be smooth or nodular
- Nonspecific; seen in spectrum of disorders
- Idiopathic invasive pachymeningitis can mimic neoplasm, aggressive infection (e.g., fungal)

Imaging Findings
General Features
- Best diagnostic sign = enhancing meninges "turn the corner" under temporal lobes in continuous line from vertex (coronal scan)
- Involves at least 75% of dural surface
- Follows inner calvarium, extends along falx and tentorium
- Can be linear or nodular, diffuse or diffuse + focal masslike
- May compress but otherwise usually spares underlying CSF cisterns, pia

CT Findings
- NECT: Isodense diffuse dural thickening
- CECT: Uniform, intense enhancement

MR Findings
- Crescentic thickened dura
  - Isointense with brain on T1WI
  - Hyperintense on T2WI (fibrosing pseudotumors may be profoundly hypointense)
  - Variable on FLAIR (usually hyperintense)
- Intense, uniform enhancement
- +/- Focal bone invasion (e.g., temporal bone)
- May involve cavernous sinus, orbit
- Can extend into spine

Hypertrophic Pachymeninges

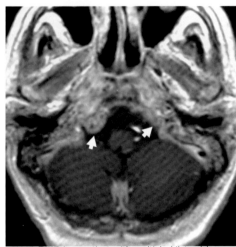

Axial post-contrast T1WI in a patient with multiple bilateral lower cranial nerve palsies shows diffuse dural thickening (arrows) with skull base invasion. Biopsy showed idiopathic invasive cranial pachymeningitis (courtesy N. Miller).

Differential Diagnosis
Subdural Hematoma (Chronic)
- May contain loculated foci of old hemorrhage
- May calcify

Intracranial Hypotension
- "Slumping" midbrain, tonsillar herniation
- Dural venous engorgement

Neoplasm
- Metastasis (adjacent skull lesions common)
- "En plaque" meningioma (may invade bone, cause hyperostosis)

Pathology
General
- Etiology-Pathogenesis
  - Congenital (mucopolysaccharidoses)
  - Iatrogenic (surgery, shunt; post-LP meningeal enhancement is rare and should be diagnosis of exclusion)
  - Trauma (cSDH, intracranial hypotension)
  - Infection (TB, HTLV-1; indolent infections such as pseudomonas, syphilis, rhinoscleroma, fungal disorders may also invade bone)
  - Inflammatory (rheumatoid, sarcoid, Wegener's, pseudotumor)
  - Neoplasm (meningiomatosis, lymphoma, metastasis)
  - Hematologic (monoclonal plasma cell hyperplasia, extramedullary hematopoiesis)
  - Other (fibrosing inflammatory pseudotumors, fibrosclerosis)
  - Idiopathic (+/- bone invasion)

Gross Pathologic or Surgical Features
- Diffuse dural thickening

Hypertrophic Pachymeninges

Microscopic Features
- Extensive meningeal fibrosis
- +/- Inflammatory cells (usually lymphocytes, plasma cells)
- May have multinucleated giant cells
- May show foci of necrosis
- Idiopathic cases show no bacteria, fungi, neoplasia

Clinical Issues
Presentation
- Headache (most common)
- Cranial neuropathy
  - Progressive sensorineural hearing loss
  - Hoarseness
  - Optic neuropathy +/- Tolosa-Hunt syndrome
- Diabetes insipidus

Natural History
- Variable course
  - Some are benign, require no treatment
  - Others have sustained remission with steroids
  - Can relapse with or without steroid dependence

Treatment & Prognosis
- Specific diagnosis may require biopsy
- Corticosteroid therapy

Selected References
1. Hatano N et al: Idiopathic hypertrophic cranial pachymeningitis: Clinicoradiological spectrum and therapeutic options. Neurosurg 45: 1336-44, 1999
2. Meltzer CC et al: MR imaging of the meninges. Part I. Normal anatomic features and nonneoplastic disease. Radiol 201: 297-308, 1996
3. Fukui MB et al: MR imaging of the meninges. Part II. Neoplastic disease. Radiol 201: 605-12, 1996

VENTRICLES AND CISTERNS

Cysts (Normal Variants)

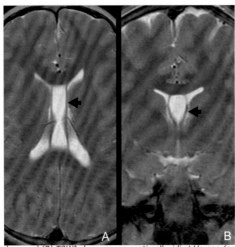

Axial (A) and coronal (B) T2WI show cavum septi pellucidi et Vergae (arrows). Note the "finger-like" posterior extension of CSF between the lateral ventricles on the axial scan (A).

Key Facts
- Cystic dilations of normal midline CSF cavities
  - Cavum septi pellucidi (CSP)
  - Cavum Vergae (CV)
  - Cavum velum interpositum (CVI)
- All are common in premature/term infants
- Normally regress but may persist as normal variants
- Occasionally enlarge, may cause mass effect (+/- symptoms)

Imaging Findings
General Features
- Best diagnostic sign = CSP/CV elongated finger-shaped; CVI triangular
CT Findings
- NECT (axial)
  - CSP
    - Leaves of septum pellucidum bowed laterally
    - > 1 cm
    - +/- Foramen of Monro obstruction, hydrocephalus
  - CV
    - CSP almost always present (CV = posterior continuation of CSP)
    - Between corpus callosum, fornix
    - Runs anteroposteriorly from rostrum/genu to splenium
  - CVI
    - Triangular-shaped
    - Doesn't extend anteriorly to foramen of Monro
    - CSP absent
- CECT: Don't enhance

Cysts (Normal Variants)

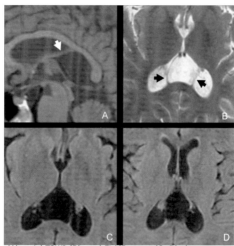

Sagittal T1- (A), axial T2WI (B), and FLAIR scans (C, D) show a cyst of the cavum velum interpositum (B, arrows). Note triangular shape on axial view. The cyst bows the fornix up (A, arrow) and displaces the ICV, pineal gland inferiorly.

MR Findings
- Sagittal
  - CSP + CV = between corpus callosum above, ICVs below (bowed downwards); doesn't stop at foramen of Monro
  - CVI = between fornix above, ICVs and 3rd ventricle below; stops at foramen of Monro
- Variable size; like CSF on all sequences (suppresses on FLAIR)

Differential Diagnosis
Arachnoid, Ependymal Cysts
- May be indistinguishable
Epidermoid Cyst
- Doesn't suppress with FLAIR
- DWI shows restriction

Pathology
General
- General Path Comments
  - CSP, CV aren't lined by ependyma, don't contain choroid
    - Precise etiology of cystic expansion is unknown
    - May be related to pressure gradient involving septal capillaries, veins
- Embryology
  - Septum pellucidum (SP)
    - Membranous structure between corpus callosum, fornix
    - Invariably cystic in fetus
    - Closes in rostral direction at 6 gestational months
    - Usually obliterated at birth
  - Velum interpositum (VI)

- Infolding of pia (tela choroidea) in transverse fissure
- Between fornix (above), roof of 3rd ventricle, thalami below
- Creates a cistern that contains the ICVs, pChA
- Etiology-Pathogenesis-Pathophysiology
  - CSP, CV form if fetal SP fails to obliterate
    - CSP is not the "fifth ventricle"
    - CV is not the "sixth ventricle"
  - CVI = dilatation of the VI
- Epidemiology
  - CSP
    - Present in 100% of premature, 85% term infants
    - Reported from as low as 1% up to 15%-20% of adults
    - Often occurs without CV
  - CV
    - 100% at fetal age 6 months, 30% term
    - <1% of adults
    - Rarely (if ever) occurs without CSP
  - CVI: Common in early infancy, rare in adults

Gross Pathologic, Surgical Features
- CSP, CV may/may not communicate with ventricles
- VI is pial-lined CSF-filled space that communicates directly with quadrigeminal cistern

Microscopic Features
- CSP, CV may contain glial cells, scattered neurons

Staging or Grading Criteria
- Shaw and Ellsworth classification for CSP, CV
  - Asymptomatic, incidental cavum (communicating or not)
  - Symptomatic, pathological, noncommunicating cavum
    - Simple and uncomplicated
    - Complicated by other lesions

Clinical Issues
Presentation
- Usually asymptomatic, incidental
- Headache = most common but relationship to cyst unclear
- May remain asymptomatic even if mass effect present
- Expanding CSP may have visual, behavioral, autonomic symptoms

Natural History
- CSP begins to regress at fetal age 8 months

Treatment & Prognosis
- Symptomatic cysts usually drained/shunted

Selected References
1. Sencer A et al: CSF dynamics of the cava septi pellucidi and vergae. J Neurosurg 94: 127-9, 2001
2. Chen C-Y et al: Sonographic characteristics of the cavum velum interpositum. AJNR 19: 1631-35, 1998
3. Van Tassel P, Cure JK: Nonneoplastic intracranial cysts and cystic lesions. Sem US, CT, MRI 16: 186-211, 1995

Obstructive Hydrocephalus (OH)

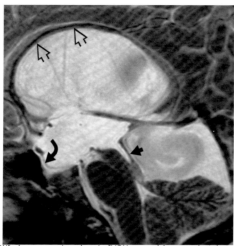

Sagittal T2WI shows massive chronic IVOH caused by aqueductal stenosis (black arrow). Note massively enlarged lateral ventricles, thinned corpus callosum (open arrows), 3rd ventricle herniated into sella (curved arrow)(courtesy J. Rees).

Key Facts
- Large ventricles without loss/dysgenesis of brain tissue
- Due to absolute/relative CSF obstruction (mismatch between formation, absorption)
- Intra- (IVOH), extraventricular (EVOH) hydrocephalus = obstruction before, beyond foramina of Luschka, Magendie
- Can be acute (aOH) or chronic (cOH)

Imaging Findings
General Features
- Global/focally enlarged ventricle(s) +/- elevated ICP
- Best diagnostic sign (aOH) = "ballooned" ventricles with indistinct ("blurred") margins

CT Findings
- NECT (aOH)
  - Large ventricles
    - Bifrontal horn diameter/intracranial diameter > .33
    - Acute frontal horn angle (< 100°)
    - Temporal horn width > 3 mm
  - Indistinct/blurred margins, periventricular low density "halo"
  - Basal cisterns, sulci compressed/obliterated
- CECT
  - Negative (if OH secondary to neoplasm, tumor may enhance)

MR Findings
- Sagittal T1WI
  - Lateral ventricles enlarged
  - Corpus callosum thinned, stretched upward
  - Fornix, ICV displaced downward
  - 3rd ventricle often enlarged, herniated into expanded sella

Obstructive Hydrocephalus (OH)

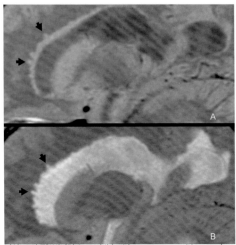

Sagittal PD- (A) and T2WI (B) in a child with nausea, vomiting, and posterior fossa mass (not shown). Acute obstructive hydrocephalus with transependymal CSF flow is illustrated (arrows).

- T2WI
  - "Fingers" of CSF-like hyperintensity extend outwards from ventricles into brain
    - Most striking around ventricular horns
  - Disturbed/turbulent CSF flow in ventricles
  - Absent aqueductal "flow void" common
  - Corpus callosum may appear hyperintense
- Contrast-enhanced T1WI
  - Hydrocephalus can induce leptomeningeal vascular stasis, mimic meningitis, metastases!

Other Modality Findings
- Cardiac-gated cine-MR
  - May show no significant CSF flow in aqueduct
- Isotope cisternography may show ventricular reflux, stasis (EVOH)

Imaging Recommendations
- 3-D constructive interference in steady state (CISS) decreases CSF flow artifact, allows better delineation of ventricular contour, septa
- Cardiac-gated phase-contrast cine MR

Differential Diagnosis

Ventricular Enlargement Secondary to Parenchymal Loss
- Age-related; ischemia/infarction; trauma; infection; toxic
- Obtuse frontal angle (>110°)
- Diffuse/focal enlargement of sulci, cisterns

Normal Pressure Hydrocephalus (see "NPH" Diagnosis)
- Progressive dementia, gait disturbance, incontinence
- Ventricular dilation with normal CSF pressure
- Sulci normal/minimally enlarged
- Increased CSF displacement through aqueduct

Obstructive Hydrocephalus (OH)

cOH ("Arrested" or "Compensated" Hydrocephalus)
- Large ventricles, normal CSF pressure
- No periventricular halo

Long-Standing Overt Ventriculomegaly in Adults (LOVA)
- Early childhood onset or long-standing progression of hydrocephalus into adulthood
- Markedly enlarged ventricles, high ICP

Pathology

General
- General Path Comments
  - Imbalance between CSF production, absorption
- Genetics
  - Cell adhesion molecule L1 (L1CAM) only gene recognized to cause human hydrocephalus
- Etiology-Pathogenesis
  - Classic theory
    - Obstruction to CSF flow develops
    - CSF production continues, ventricular fluid pressure increases
    - Ventricles expand, compress adjacent parenchyma
    - Stretching may rupture/open ependymal cell junctions
    - Periventricular interstitial fluid increases
  - New: Overexpression of some growth factors (TGF), mutated Otx2 (head organizer during morphogenesis) reported
  - Rare: More CSF produced than can be absorbed ("over-production" hydrocephalus; occurs with CPP, villous hyperplasia)
- Epidemiology
  - Most common neurosurgical procedure in children= CSF shunting

Gross Pathologic or Surgical Features
- Focal/generalized ventricular enlargement

Microscopic Features
- Increased periventricular extracellular space

Clinical Issues

Presentation
- Headache, papilledema

Natural History
- Usually progressive unless treated

Treatment & Prognosis
- CSF diversion (shunt), endoscopic Rx

Selected References
1. Aleman J et al: Value of constructive interference in steady-state, three-dimensional, Fourier transformation magnetic resonance imaging for the neuroendoscopic treatment of hydrocephalus and intracranial cysts. Neurosurg 48: 1291-6, 2001
2. Pena A et al: Effects of brain ventricular shape on periventricular biomechanics: A finite-element analysis. Neurosurg 45: 107-18, 2000
3. Oi S et al: Pathophysiology of long-standing overt ventriculomegaly in adults. J Neurosurg 92: 933-40, 2000

Normal Pressure Hydro (NPH)

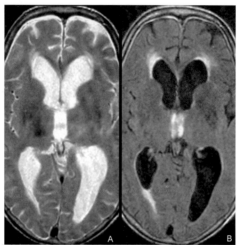

79-year-old demented female with T2WI (A) and FLAIR (B) scans showing large ventricles, normal sulci. Aqueductal stroke volume was 236 μL, suggesting NPH. Ventricular shunting produced dramatic improvement.

Key Facts
- Heterogeneous syndrome (classic clinical triad = dementia, gait apraxia, urinary incontinence)
- Ventriculomegaly + normal CSF pressure, altered CSF dynamics
- Diagnostic challenge = identify shunt-responsive NPH

Imaging Findings
General Features
- Best diagnostic sign = combination of large ventricles, Sylvian fissures + normal hippocampus, sulci

CT Findings
- NECT: Ventriculomegaly with rounded frontal horns

MR Findings
- Increased ventricular volume
- Large frontal, temporal horns without hippocampal atrophy
- Enlarged basal cisterns, Sylvian fissures; sulci normal
- Corpus callosum bowed upwards (may be impinged by falx)
- Aqueductal "flow void" sign
  - Present in some cases on PD, conventional SE sequences
  - May be reduced if flow-compensation, FSE techniques used
  - Controversial indicator of shunt-responsiveness
- 50%-60% have periventricular, deep white matter lesions on T2WI
  - More frequent, severe compared to age-matched controls
  - Correlates with poor outcome after shunting

Other Modality Findings
- CSF flow studies to detect increased velocity ("hyperdynamic" flow)
  - Cardiac-gated 2D-FISP
  - Aqueduct stroke volume > 42 μL reported to correlated with good response to shunt
  - Some patients with normal CSF flow values also improve

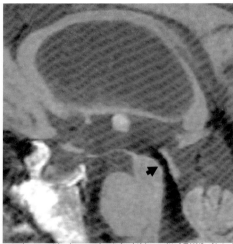

Elderly demented man with abnormal gait had this sagittal T1WI. Note large lateral, third ventricles with prominent aqueductal "flow void" (arrow). Findings suggestive (but not pathognomonic for) NPH. Incidental colloid cyst is also present.

- Isotope cisternography demonstrates ventricular flow
- SPECT, PET: Hypoperfusion, decreased metabolism common
- ICP monitoring: Wave amplitude > 9mm Hg correlates with post-shunt cognitive improvement

Imaging Recommendations
- MR with CSF flow studies

Differential Diagnosis
Alzheimer Dementia
- Dementia out of proportion to gait disturbance
- Large perihippocampal fissures, small hippocampi

Multi-Infarct Dementia
- Multiple infarcts on imaging

Pathology
General
- General Path Comments
  - Pathogenesis of NPH poorly understood
- Etiology-Pathogenesis
  - 50% idiopathic; 50% other (e.g., SAH)
  - Age-related changes in CSF formation/absorption include increased resistance to CSF outflow
    - May be exacerbated in NPH
  - NPH: Reduced CBF, altered CSF resorption without increased CSF pressure
    - Brain expands in systole, causes CSF displacement
    - Loss of parenchymal compliance, altered viscoelastic properties of ventricular wall
    - Increased interstitial fluid
    - Pulsation pressure directed toward ventricles

- "Water-hammer" effect
- May be further complicated by microangiopathy (including venous compromise), atrophy
- Epidemiology
  - Accounts for approximately 0.5-5% of dementias
  - Most common in patients > 60y
  - M > F

Gross Pathologic or Surgical Features
- Enlarged ventricles, normal CSF pressure

Microscopic Features
- Arachnoid fibrosis in 50%
- Cerebral parenchyma
  - Almost 50% show no significant parenchymal pathology
  - 20% have neurofibrillary tangles, other changes of AD
  - 10% arteriosclerosis, ischemic encephalomalacia

Clinical Issues

Presentation
- Dementia, gait disturbance, incontinence

Natural History
- Progressive decline in cognitive function

Treatment & Prognosis
- Variable outcome (25%-80% of shunted patients improve)

Selected References
1. Czosnyka M et al: Age dependence of cerebrospinal pressure-volume compensation in patients with hydrocephalus. J Neurosurg 94: 482-6, 2001
2. Parkkola RK et al: Cerebrospinal fluid flow in patients with dilated ventricles studied with MR imaging. Eur Radiol 10: 1442-6, 2000
3. Bech RA et al: Frontal brain and leptomeningeal biopsy specimens correlated with CSF outflow resistance and B-wave activity in patients suspected of NPH. Neurosurg 40: 497-502, 1997

CSF Shunts and Complications

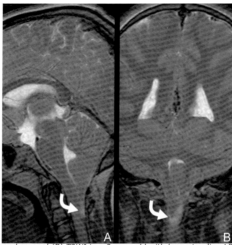

Sagittal (A) and coronal (B) T2WI in a 9-year-old with long-standing LP shunt show severe acquired tonsillar herniation (arrows).

Key Facts
- Many different pediatric disorders may necessitate CSF diversion
- Shunting obstructed ventricles restores vascular compliance ⇒ restores normal trans-parenchymal drainage patterns
- Common complications include shunt obstruction/breakage, infection, overdrainage
- Non-compliant ventricle syndrome = older child (shunted in infancy), small ventricles + intermittent signs of shunt obstruction

Imaging Findings
General Features
- Image to define site (intra-, extraventricular), etiology of block
- Best diagnostic sign = dilated ventricles + fluid/edema "blurring" margin around valve/ventricles
CT Findings
- NECT
  - Ventricular dilatation (diffuse or loculated)
  - Transependymal CSF egress ("blurred" ventricles)
  - Non-compliant ventricle syndrome
    - Ventricles may appear normal/small even if shunt is malfunctioning!
    - Can be caused by shunt-induced sutural ossification
  - +/- Subdural fluid (overdrainage in younger patients)
  - Previous studies for comparison needed for best diagnosis
- CECT
  - +/- Ependymal enhancement
  - May identify other abnormalities (meningitis, neoplasm, etc)
MR Findings
- "Fingers" of CSF extending into periventricular WM common
- 2D PC MR flow studies may identify obstruction (e.g., aqueduct)

CSF Shunts and Complications

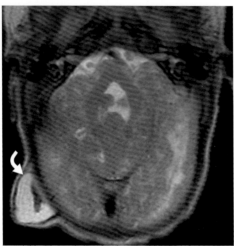

Axial T2WI in a child with cerebellar dysplasia and blocked shunt shows a large fluid collection (curved arrow) under the scalp around the reservoir.

Other Modality Findings
- Plain films: Evaluate shunt continuity/integrity
  - Shunt fractures/separation (13%)
  - Shunt migration (rare = bowel perforation)
- Contrast shuntogram: Defines site of blockage (rarely performed)
- Radionuclide studies: Rarely performed

Imaging Recommendations
- Most important: Baseline CT/MR following shunt insertion!
- Follow-up at 1y, then as needed

Differential Diagnosis

Normal Post-Shunt
- Clinical findings (symptomatic)
- Compare to baseline

Increased Intracranial Pressure
- Small/effaced sulci, cisterns
- Small, "slit-like" ventricles may occur with non-compliant ventricle syndrome, chronic overdrainage

Pathology

General
- General Path Comments
  - Infected shunts 5%-10%
  - Ventricular loculation 6%
  - Overshunting 3% (subdural effusions/hematomas)
- Etiology-Pathogenesis-Pathophysiology
  - Each shunt, valve/device carries own set of complications
    - VP (ventriculoperitoneal) ⇒ abdominal complications
    - VA (ventriculoatrial) ⇒ shunt nephritis, cor pulmonale
    - LP (lumboperitoneal) ⇒ arachnoiditis, cerebellar tonsillar herniation, high migration rate

CSF Shunts and Complications

- - Internal 3rd ventricle to spinal SAS (Lapras catheter) $\Rightarrow$ no external access, no way to check flow
  - Shuntless CSF diversion: 3rd ventriculostomy, 4th ventricle outlet fenestration $\Rightarrow$ 70% patency
  - Anti-siphon devices $\Rightarrow$ obstruction by capsule formation
  - Flanged catheters increased risk of proximal occlusion
  - Programmable shunt $\Rightarrow$ remember to reprogram after MRI
  - One piece shunt $\Rightarrow$ decreased obstruction rate but increased slit ventricle/SDH rate
  - Ventriculopleural if peritoneum contaminated or cardiac complicated, but $\Rightarrow$ pleural effusion
  - o Ependymal "scar" may reduce capability of ventricle to expand
- Epidemiology
  - o CSF shunts in USA = 125,000
  - o Shunt malfunction
    - 20%-40% at 1y, 80% at 12y follow-up

Gross Pathologic, Surgical Features
- Transventricular ependymal adhesions
Microscopic Features
- Gliosis along tract

Clinical Issues
Presentation
- Shunt failure
  - o Common: H/A, N&V, drowsiness
  - o Infants: Bulging fontanel, increased head circumference
Natural History
- Most shunts eventually fail; failure induces further failure
- 50% multiple revisions, progressively shorter intervals
Treatment & Prognosis
- Lengthen distal shunt as child grows
- Change intraventricular component/valve if proximal obstruction
- Alter pressure valve if over/under-draining
- Subtemporal decompression/3rd ventriculostomy for non-compliant ventricle syndrome
- Outcome largely depends on initial pathology that required shunting

Selected References
1. Drake JM et al: CSF shunts 50 years on –past, present and future. Childs Nerv Syst 16: 800-4,2000
2. Lee TT et al: Unique clinical presentation of pediatric shunt malfunction. Pediatr Neurosurg 30: 122-6,1999
3. Tuli S et al: Risk factors for repeated CSF shunt failures in pediatric patients with hydrocephalus. J Neurosurg 92:31-38, 2000

Enlarged Subarachnoid Spaces

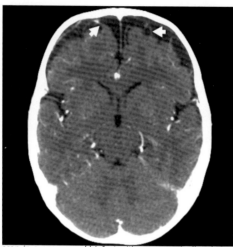

Axial CECT scan in a one year old infant with macrocrania (head circumference > 95th percentile) shows very prominent bifrontal extra-axial fluid spaces that are identical in attenuation to CSF. Note several linear enhancing structures (cortical veins, arrows) cross the spaces. The underlying gyri appear normal.

Key Facts
- Idiopathic enlargement of SAS common, normal ≅ 3 – 8 months age
- Likely due to immature CSF drainage pathways
- Self-limited; resolves without therapy by 12-24 months

Imaging Findings
General Features
- Best diagnostic sign = enlarged SAS **and** ↑ head circumference (> 95%)

CT Findings
- NECT
  - ≥ 5mm widening bifrontal/anterior interhemispheric SAS
  - ↑ Cisterns (especially suprasellar/chiasmatic)
  - Sulci generally normal (especially posteriorly)
  - Posterior fossa normal
  - Mild ↑ ventricles (66%)
- CECT: Demonstrates veins traverse SAS

MR Findings
- Single layer of fluid (SAS) **with** traversing vessels
- SAS isointense with CSF on all sequences

Other Modality Findings
- Fetal MRI: Seen in fetus with posterior distribution fluid/ventricular prominence due to positioning (usually frontal prominence after birth due to child lying on back for scan)
- Color doppler sonography: Veins traverse SAS
- Isotope cisternography: Accumulation of CSF in 4th and lateral ventricles similar to extraventricular hydrocephalus

Imaging Recommendations
- Doppler sonography: Documents veins traversing SAS

Enlarged Subarachnoid Spaces

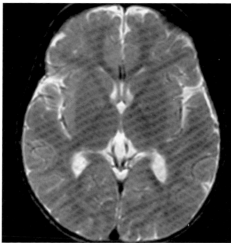

Same case as previous figure. Follow-up axial T2WI obtained at age 2 shows the prominent extra-axial spaces have disappeared. The subarachnoid spaces and ventricles appear normal. The myelin pattern is normal for this age. The CECT scan at 1 year represented benign enlargement of the subarachnoid spaces in infancy.

- MRI: Exclude chronic subdural collections
- After diagnosis, best followup = tape measure, **not** imaging!

Differential Diagnosisf
Atrophy
- Small head (circumference measurement critical!)
- Benign SAS enlargement has large head

Extraventricular Obstructive Hydrocephalus (EVOH)
- Often hemorrhagic/post inflammatory/neoplastic
- If present, extra-axial collection not = CSF
- Can mimic NAT (see "Non-accidental Trauma" diagnosis)
  - Predisposition to bleed with minor trauma controversial
    - Possible if SAS larger than 6 mm

Pathology
General
- Etiology-Pathogenesis-Pathophysiology
  - Immature CSF drainage pathways
    - CSF primarily drained via extracellular space $\Rightarrow$ capillaries
    - Pacchionian granulations don't mature until $\approx$18 months
    - Pacchionian granulations are then displaced into veins (as Starling-type resistors)
    - Regulate pulse pressure/venous drainage CSF when fontanelles close
    - Benign SAS enlargement usually resolves at that time
- Epidemiology
  - 80% male

Enlarged Subarachnoid Spaces

Gross Pathologic, Surgical Features
- Deep/ prominent but otherwise normal-appearing SAS
- No pathologic membranes
- Clear CSF

Microscopic Features
- N/A

Clinical Issues

Presentation
- **No** signs of ↑ICP
- Family history of benign macrocephaly common
- Head circumference > 95%
- Mild developmental delay in 50% (motor >language)

Natural History
- Spontaneous resolution of spaces and symptoms by 12-24 months
- Normal outcome (developmental delay resolves as prominent SAS resolves)
- Macrocephaly often persists

Treatment & Prognosis
- No treatment necessary
- ↑ SAS ⇒ ↑ suture/calvarial malleability/compliance ⇒ predispose to posterior plagiocephaly

Selected References
1. Greitz D et al: The pathogenesis and hemodynamics of hydrocephalus: Proposal for a new understanding. IJNR 3:367-75,1997
2. Prassopoulos P et al: The size of the intra-and extraventricular CSF compartments in children with idiopathic benign widening of the frontal subarachnoid space. Neuroradiology 37:418-21,1995
3. Freide RL. Ch. 20: Hydrocephalus-special pathology. In: Developmental neuropathology, 2nd ed. Springer-Verlag, Berlin, 1989

METABOLIC WHITE MATTER, DEGENERATIVE DISEASE

Normal Aging Brain

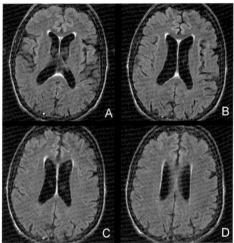

Normal aging brain. (A-D) Axial FLAIR scans in an intellectually normal 65-year-old male show prominent sulci ventricles with high signal intensity periventricular "rims" and "caps" (around bodies, frontal horns).

Key Facts
- Broad spectrum of "normal" on imaging studies in elderly
- Brain shrinks, CSF spaces increase
- Selective atrophy of white (not gray) matter predominates!
- Can't predict cognitive function from standard CT/MR

Imaging Findings
General Features
- Brain tissue decreases, CSF volume increases
  - ○ Reflects WM volume loss
  - ○ Volume of WM hyperintensities doesn't contribute significantly
- Metabolic alterations common
  - ○ Global and regional changes in CBF
- Best diagnostic clue = thin periventricular high-signal rim without white matter hyperintensities ("successfully aging brain")
CT Findings
- NECT
  - ○ Enlarged ventricles, widened cortical sulci
  - ○ Patchy/confluent periventricular low densities common
MR Findings
- PD, FLAIR: Smooth, thin hyperintense periventricular rim normal
- T2 hyperintensity
  - ○ Focal/confluent periventricular WMHs
    - ▪ Number, size increase after 50y; nearly universal (normal) after 65
    - ▪ Only rough correlation with cognitive function
    - ▪ Significant overlap with dementias
  - ○ "Infarctlike" lesions
    - ▪ Seen in 1/3 of asymptomatic patients >65y
    - ▪ 70% < 10 mm
    - ▪ Mostly in basal ganglia, thalami

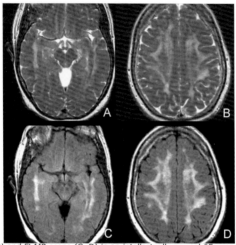

T2WI (A, B) and FLAIR scans (C, D) in an intellectually normal 65-year-old woman. Note striking confluent periventricular and deep white matter hyperintensity.

- ▪ Probably represent clinically silent lacunar infarcts
- T2 shortening
  - ○ "Black line" in visual, motor/sensory cortex common, normal in older patients
  - ○ Ferric iron deposition
    - ▪ Normal in globus pallidus (GP) normal
    - ▪ Increases in caudate/putamen and may = GP by eighth decade
    - ▪ Abnormal in thalamus
- T2*: "Black dots" in patients >60y with co-existing WMHs
  - ○ **Not** normal
  - ○ Long-standing hypertension, amyloid angiopathy

Other Modality Findings
- MRS: Decreased %NAA, NAA:Cho, NAA:Cr
- DWI: Small but significant increased water diffusibility
  - ○ ADC increases
  - ○ Decreased anisotropy on diffusion tensor imaging
- PET: Decreased pre-/postsynaptic dopamine markers in basal ganglia
- ^{99m}Tc-HMPAO SPECT, Xe-133 inhalation show regional, global reduction in CBF

Imaging Recommendations
- MR: Include T2* on all patients >60y

Differential Diagnosis

Mild Cognitive Impairment (MCI)
- Overlap with normal on standard imaging studies
- Higher **calculated** hippocampal ADCs (not visible)
- Subtle hypoperfusion, hypometabolism in perihippocampal regions, cingulum, thalamus

Alzheimer Dementia (AD)
- Striking temporoparietal hypometabolism, hypoperfusion

- Striking volume loss in hippocampi, entorhinal cortex

Subcortical Microvascular Encephalopathy
- Numerous WMHs (overlap with normal)
- Clinical picture of vascular dementia

Pathology

General
- Etiology-Pathogenesis
  - Old view of aging: Substantial cortical neuronal loss with age
  - New: Predominant neuroanatomic changes =
    - White matter alterations, subcortical neuronal loss
    - Reduction in cell size > cell number
  - Neuronal dysfunction rather than loss of neurons/synapses
- Epidemiology
  - WMHs correlate with age, silent stroke, hypertension, female gender

Gross Pathologic or Surgical Features
- Widened sulci, large ventricles

Microscopic Features
- Decreased myelinated fibers in subcortical WM
- Increased extracellular space, gliosis
- Iron deposition in globus pallidus, putamen
- WM capillaries lose pericytes, have thinner endothelium

Clinical Issues

Presentation
- Normal cognitive function
- Mild cognitive impairment (MCI) correlates with subsequent increase in developing AD

Natural History
- Parenchymal volume decreases, CSF spaces increase progressively
- WMHs progressively increase with age

Selected References
1. Angelie E et al: Regional differences and metabolic changes in normal aging of the human brain: Proton MR spectroscopic imaging study. AJNR 22: 119-27, 2001
2. Nusbaum AO et al: Regional and global changes in cerebral diffusion with normal aging. AJNR 22: 136-42, 2001
3. Guttmann CRG et al: White matter changes with normal aging. Neurology 50: 972-8, 1998

Microvascular Disease

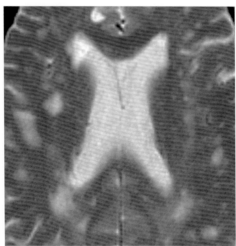

Axial T2WI in an intellectually normal 72-year-old male with long-standing hypertension, diabetes and generalized ASVD shows multifocal white matter hyperintensities characteristic of atherosclerotic microvasculopathy.

Key Facts
- Significance of white matter hyperintensities (WMHs) controversial
- WMHs generally related to cerebrovascular risk factors (hypertension, age, hypercholesterolemia, diabetes, etc.)
- Spectrum of histopathologic correlates

Imaging Findings
General Features
- Common in periventricular/deep WM, basal ganglia
- Best diagnostic clue = white matter rarefaction on CT; patchy/ confluent hyperintensity on PD/ T2WI/ FLAIR

CT Findings
- NECT: Multifocal/confluent ill-defined hypodense areas =/> 5mm
- CECT: No enhancement

MR Findings
- Ill-defined hyperintensities =/> 5mm on PD/T2WI, FLAIR
- +/- "Black dots" on T2* (similar to chronic HTN, amyloid)
- +/- Generalized atrophy (large ventricles, sulci)
- Extensive/confluent lesions found in 2%-6% of normal elderly!

Other Modality Findings
- MRS: Reduced NAA, NAA/Cr
- PET/SPECT: In absence of atrophy, rCBF/rMRGlu usually normal

Imaging Recommendations
- MR (include FLAIR, GRE sequences)

Differential Diagnosis
Age-Related White Matter Changes
- Significant overlap between normal, demented elderly
- Normal rCBF

Microvascular Disease

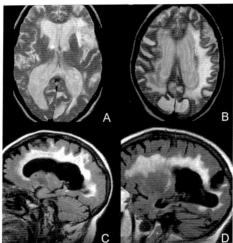

Axial T2WI (A, B) and FLAIR scans (C, D) in an elderly demented patient with clinical diagnosis of Binswanger's disease show bilateral but asymmetric confluent periventricular WM hyperintensity. Subcortical atherosclerotic encephalopathy. Multiple cortical infarcts are also present.

Perivascular (Virchow-Robin) Spaces
- Variable size, well-delineated
- Most common around anterior commissure, deep WM
- Signal, attenuation like CSF

Lacunar Infarcts
- Seen in 1/3 of healthy elderly (often asymptomatic)
- 3-10 mm, sharply delineated, hyperintense on PD
- Most (almost 80%) in deep nuclear regions (caudate, lentiform nuclei, internal capsule, thalamus)

Vascular Dementia (VaD)
- Cognitive impairment
  - Multi-infarct dementia (MID)
  - Subcortical arteriosclerotic encephalopathy ("Binswanger" type vascular dementia)
    - Clinical (not imaging) diagnosis
    - Long-standing HTN, progressive decline in mental function, gait disturbances, with or without minor strokes
- Large, small infarcts
- Decreased rCBF

Pathology
General
- General Path Comments
  - "Microangiopathy-related cerebral damage" = WMHs, lacunar infarcts
  - WMHs on imaging don't always have pathologic correlates
- Genetics
  - General risk factors for peripheral/cerebral vascular diseases
    - APOE ε4 alleles
    - Angiotensinogen gene promoter

Microvascular Disease

- o Cerebral autosomal dominant arteriopathy with subcortical infarct and leukoencephalopathy (CADASIL)
    - Notch3 mutations
- Etiology-Pathogenesis
  - o Hypertensive occlusive disease of small penetrating arteries
    - Results in lacunar infarcts, deep white matter lesions
  - o Venous collagenosis (controversial)
- Epidemiology
  - o WMHs almost universal after 65y
  - o Lacunar infarcts in 1/3 of asymptomatic healthy patients >65y
  - o Vascular dementia (VaD) third most common cause of dementia (after AD, Lewy body disease), accounts for 15% of cases

Gross Pathologic or Surgical Features
- N/A

Microscopic Features
- Normal age-related changes (see "Normal Aging Brain")
- Imaging WMHs have spectrum of histopathologic correlates
  - o Degenerated myelin (myelin "pallor")
  - o Axonal loss, increased intra-/extracellular fluid
  - o Gliosis, spongiosis
  - o Arteriosclerosis, small vessel occlusions

Staging or Grading Criteria
- European Task Force on Age-Related White Matter Changes
- ARWMC Rating Scale for MRI and CT (for ill-defined lesions =/> 5mm)
  - o White matter lesions
    - 0 = No lesions (including symmetrical caps, bands)
    - 1 = Focal lesions
    - 2 = Beginning confluence of lesions
    - 3 = Diffuse involvement, with or without U fibers
  - o Basal ganglia lesions
    - 0 = No lesions
    - 1 = 1 focal lesion (=/> 5 mm)
    - 2 = > 1 focal lesion
    - 3 = Confluent lesions

Clinical Issues
Presentation
- Broad range (normal to minimal cognitive impairment to demented)
Natural History
- Little known

Selected References
1. Wahlund LO et al: A new rating scale for age-related white matter changes applicable to MRI and CT. Stroke 32: 1318-22, 2001
2. Schmidt H et al: Angiotensinogen gene promoter haplotype and microangiopathy-related cerebral damage. Stroke 32: 405-412, 2001
3. Yao H et al: Cerebral blood flow in nondemented elderly subjects with extensive deep white matter lesions on MRI. J Stroke Cerebrovasc Dis 9: 172-5, 2000

Cerebral Angiopathy (CAA)

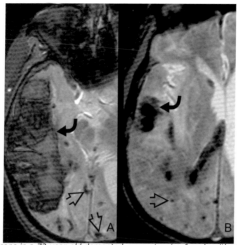

Axial T2* scans in a 72-year-old demented, normotensive female with spontaneous lobar hemorrhage (curved arrows) also shows multifocal "black dots" (open arrows). Cerebral amyloid angiopathy (CAA).

Key Facts
- CAA is common cause of "spontaneous" lobar hemorrhage in elderly (see "Primary Intracerebral Hemorrhage")
- CAA common in elderly patient with dementia (e.g., Alzheimer)

Imaging Findings
General Features
- Superficial hemorrhages involve cortex, subcortical WM
- Best diagnostic sign = normotensive demented patient with
  - Lobar hemorrhage(s), different ages
  - Multifocal "black dots"

CT Findings
- NECT
  - Patchy or confluent cortical/subcortical hematoma with irregular borders, surrounding edema
  - Rare: Gyriform Ca++
- CECT
  - No enhancement

MR Findings
- T1WI
  - Lobar hematoma (signal varies with age of clot)
  - Generalized atrophy common (prominent ventricles, sulci)
- T2WI
  - Acute hematoma; 1/3 have old hemorrhages (lobar, petechial)
  - Focal or patchy/confluent WM disease in nearly 70%
  - Fare: Nonhemorrhagic diffuse encephalopathy with confluent WM hyperintensities
- T2*
  - Multifocal "black dots"
- Rare: CAA can cause focal, nonhemorrhagic mass(es), enhance, mimic neoplasm!

Cerebral Angiopathy (CAA)

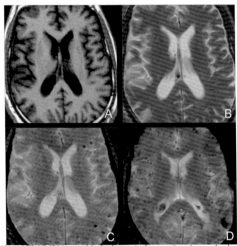

Axial T1- (A) and T2WI (B) in an elderly demented normotensive male show prominent sulci, ventricles. (C, D) GRE scans show innumerable "black dots." Biopsy showed CAA. (Courtesy R.Kalnins).

Other Modality Findings
- DSA: Normal or avascular mass effect

Imaging Recommendations
- Include T2*-weighted sequence in patients >60y

Differential Diagnosis

Hypertensive Microhemorrhages
- History of chronic HTN
- Deep structures (basal ganglia, thalami) > cortex, subcortical WM
- Often Co-Exist With CAA

Ischemic Stroke With Microhemorrhage
- Multifocal hemosiderin deposits (10%-15% of patients with ischemic stroke)
- Hemorrhagic lacunar infarcts

Multiple Vascular Malformations
- Cavernous, capillary malformations
  - Look for "locules" of blood with fluid-fluid levels
  - Capillary hemangiomas may show faint, "brush-like" enhancement

Other Causes of Multifocal "Black Dots"
- Traumatic axonal injury (history, location in corpus callosum)
- Hemorrhagic metastases (may enhance, location at gray-white junction)

Pathology

General
- General Path Comments
  - CNS amyloid can cause lobar hemorrhage (most common), microangiopathy, focal "amyloidoma" (least common)
- Genetics
  - Sporadic
    - APOE4 allele associated with CAA-related hemorrhage
    - Polymorphisms in presenilin-1 gene

Cerebral Angiopathy (CAA)

- o Hereditary cerebral hemorrhage with amyloidosis
  - ▪ Autosomal dominant inheritance
  - ▪ Dutch type = mutated amyloid β precursor protein on chromosome 21
  - ▪ Other types include British, Flemish, etc.
- Etiology-Pathogenesis-Pathophysiology
  - o Amyloidosis = rare systemic disease caused by extracellular deposition of β-amyloid
  - o 10%-20% localized form, including CNS
  - o Can be idiopathic/primary or secondary/reactive (e.g., dialysis-related amyloidosis)
- Epidemiology
  - o 1% of all strokes
  - o Causes up to 15%-20% of pICH in patients > 60y
  - o Frequency of CAA in elderly
    - ▪ 27%-32% of normal elderly (autopsy)
    - ▪ 82%-88% in patients with Alzheimer disease (AD)
    - ▪ Common in Down syndrome

Gross Pathologic or Surgical Features
- Lobar hemorrhage
- Multiple small cortical hemorrhages

Microscopic Features
- Interstitial, vascular/perivascular deposits of amorphous protein
  - o Stains with Congo red
  - o Birefringent under polarized light
- Microaneurysms
- Fibrinoid necrosis
- Perivascular infiltrates
- Hyaline thickening

Clinical Issues
Presentation
- Spontaneous lobar hemorrhage
- 40% with subacute dementia/overt AD
- 2/3 normotensive; 1/3 HTN

Natural History
- Multiple, recurrent hemorrhages
- Progressive cognitive decline

Treatment & Prognosis
- Evacuate focal hematoma if patient <75y, no IVH, not parietal
- Low Glasgow Coma Scale scores, APOE4 allele adverse prognostic factors

Selected References
1. McCarron MO et al: Cerebral amyloid angiopathy-related hemorrhage. Stroke 30: 1643-6, 1999
2. Good CD et al: Amyloid angiopathy causing widespread miliary haemorrhages within the brain evident on MRI. Neuroradiol 40: 308-11, 1998
3. Chan S et al: Multifocal hypointense cerebral lesions on gradient-echo MR are associated with chronic hypertension. AJNR 17: 1821-7, 1996

Alzheimer Dementia (AD)

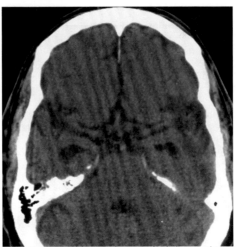

NECT scan in a patient with Alzheimer dementia (AD) diagnosed at age 59 shows prominent basal cisterns, enlarged temporal horns, atrophic medial temporal lobes with small hippocampi.

Key Facts
- AD is most common dementia/cause of cerebral atrophy in elderly
- Prevalence increases with age; up to 50% after 85y
- AD is a "taupathy" (abnormal *tau* protein accumulates, plays key role in neuronal/glial dysfunction, cell death)
- Current role of imaging in AD is to exclude "treatable" dementias, identify early-onset cases for possible innovative Rx

Imaging Findings
General Features
- Best diagnostic clue = disproportionate hippocampal volume loss

CT Findings
- Role is to rule out treatable/reversible dementias (see below)
- Shows large temporal horns, medial temporal lobe atrophy
- If no brain atrophy, patient extremely unlikely to have AD (may have "pseudodementia" caused by depression)

MR Findings
- Volume loss in entorhinal cortex, hippocampus
- Often have co-existing microvascular disease, WMHs

Other Modality Findings
- PET, SPECT
  - Regional hypometabolic areas (decreased glucose, oxygen utilization)
  - Perfusion deficits (reduced rCBF)
- MRS: Decreased NAA, increased MI
- ADC (calculated, not visual): Elevated (hippocampus, etc)

Imaging Recommendations
- Look for partially/fully reversible causes of dementia
  - Small number (up to 10%) of cases
    - Clinical/laboratory evaluation for potentially reversible causes (e.g., alcohol/drug abuse, thyroid dysfunction, depression)

Alzheimer Dementia (AD)

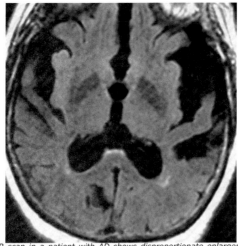

Axial FLAIR scan in a patient with AD shows disproportionate enlargement of the basal cisterns compared to the surface sulci. Note virtual absence of signal abnormality in the WM.

- o Routine CT or MR to identify other causes
    - Head injury (e.g., cSDH), mass lesion (e.g., frontal neoplasm)
    - Hydrocephalus (especially NPH)
    - Other neurodegenerative disorders (e.g., Huntington disease, degenerative diseases normally presenting in childhood)
    - Inherited or acquired white matter diseases
- Identify early AD cases for possible Rx
    - o Volumetric MR of hippocampus, entorhinal cortex
    - o Functional neuroimaging currently "not cost-effective"

Differential Diagnosis
Diffuse Lewy Body Disease (DLBD)
- Second most common dementia (10%-25% of all cases)
- 7%-30% of AD cases have concomitant Lewy bodies
- Hypometabolism of entire brain, including visual cortex/cerebellum

Frontotemporal Dementia (Lumped Under "Pick's Disease," PD)
- Heterogeneous group, accounts for 12%-20% of dementias
- Asymmetric frontal, anterior temporal atrophy

Corticobasal Degeneration
- Prominent extrapyramidal, cortical symptoms
- Severe frontoparietal atrophy

Normal Pressure Hydrocephalus (NPH)
- Gait, motor deficits common
- Severe, generalized, ventricular enlargement without disproportionate hippocampal atrophy

Pathology
General
- General Path Comments
    - o Discriminate between AD, non-AD degenerative dementias

Alzheimer Dementia (AD)

- Genetics
  - Autosomal dominant (early-onset) familial AD
    - Amyloid precursor protein (APP) gene on chromosome 21
    - 55% associated with missense point mutations of presenilin-1 gene on chromosome 14
  - Apolipoprotein E (ApoE) ε4 allele associated for increased risk, earlier age of onset
    - 60%-75% of all AD patients carry at least one copy
    - Familial AD patients often homozygous
- Etiology-Pathogenesis-Pathophysiology
  - β-amyloid (βA) aggregates seen as senile/neuritic plaques
  - β-amyloid precursor protein has pivotal role in AD
- Epidemiology
  - AD most common neurodegenerative cause of dementia
    - Accounts for 50%-75% of cases

Gross Pathologic or Surgical Features
- Shrunken gyri, widened sulci

Microscopic Features
- Neuritic plaques (NPs), neurofibrillary tangles (NFTs)
  - Tangles composed of abnormally phosphorylated **tau** protein
    - Hippocampus, neocortical/some subcortical areas
- Loss of synapses, neurons (greatest in layer 3,5)
- Amyloid angiopathy
  - βA major component of both NPs, blood vessels in AD
- Astro- and microgliosis
- Decreased fiber density in temporal white matter, with disruption/loss of axonal membranes and myelin

Clinical Issues

Presentation
- Primarily a disease of old age but autosomal dominant familial AD can present as early as 4th decade
- Initial symptom = memory impairment
- Visual variant of AD may present with impaired visuospatial skills without memory complaints

Natural History
- Chronic, progressive impairment of intellectual functions
- 65 year olds with mild cognitive impairment (MCI) subsequently diagnosed as AD at 10%-15% per year, > 50% at 5 years

Treatment & Prognosis
- New drugs for early mild/moderate AD promising

Selected References
1. Bayer TA et al: Key factors in Alzheimer's disease: ß-amyloid precursor protein processing, metabolism and intraneuronal transport. Brain Pathol 11: 1-11, 2001
2. Savoiardo M et al: Imaging dementias. Eur Radiol 11: 484-92, 2001
3. Jack CRJr et al: Hippocampal atrophy and apoliprotein E genotype are independently associated with Alzheimer's disease. Ann Neurol 43: 303-10, 1998

Alcohol and The Brain

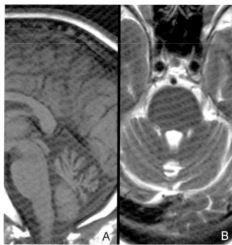

Sagittal T1- (A) and axial T2WI (B) in a chronic alcoholic show marked atrophy of the superior vermis. The supratentorial sulci and cisterns were normal.

Key Facts
- Primary (direct) effects of EtOH = neurotoxicity (cortical/cerebellar degeneration, peripheral polyneuropathy)
- Rare secondary treatable complication = Wernicke encephalopathy
- Many indirect effects of EtOH abuse (ie. trauma, malnutrition)

Imaging Findings
General Features
- Best diagnostic signs
    - EtOH: Disproportionate superior vermian atrophy
    - Methanol: Bilateral hemorrhagic putamenal necrosis
    - Wernicke's: Mammillary bodies hyperintense, +/- enhance
CT Findings
- NECT
    - EtOH: Generalized atrophy; superior vermis atrophy
    - Methanol: Bilateral hemorrhagic putamenal necrosis
MR Findings
- Chronic EtOH
    - Symmetrical enlargement of lateral ventricles
    - ↑ Size of cerebral sulci, interhemispheric/sylvian fissures
    - Dose-dependent
    - WM lesions (hyperintense on T2WI, FLAIR)
        - Bilateral periventricular, CC; isolated/confluent
        - Marchiafava-Bignami disease (mid-corpus callosum necrosis is virtually pathognomonic)
- Wernicke encephalopathy
    - T1WI: Enhancement of mamillary bodies
    - T2WI: Hyperintensity around 3rd ventricle, medial thalamus, midbrain (periaqueductal gray)
- Methanol poisoning
    - Bilateral hemorrhagic putamenal necrosis

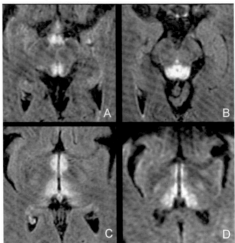

Acute Wernicke encephalopathy is illustrated. (A-C) Axial FLAIR scans show high signal intensity in the mamillary bodies, midbrain tegmentum, thalami and hypothalamus. (D) DWI shows restricted diffusion.

- o WM lesions
  - • Hemorrhagic subcortical necrosis
  - • Optic nerves often affected

Imaging Recommendations
- • NECT scan (good for complications such as SDH, coagulopathies)
- • MR for possible Wernicke encephalopathy (N.B.: Lack of imaging abnormalities does not exclude Wernicke)

Differential Diagnosis
EtOH-related vs. Nonalcoholic Atrophy
- • Multi-infarct dementia
- • Alzheimer disease
- • Malnutrition
- • Chronic trauma (repeated head blows)

Methanol vs. Other Basal Ganglia Disorders
- • Most are nonhemorrhagic
  - o Anoxic stroke
  - o CO inhalation
  - o Inherited metabolic (e.g., Wilson, Leigh, etc.)

Pathology
General
- • General Path Comments
  - o Chronic alcoholism
    - • Brain shrinkage, cortical atrophy & lifetime consumption
    - • Neuronal degeneration in anterior/superior cerebellar vermis in cases of alcoholic cerebellar degeneration
    - • 50% enlarged ventricles, sulci (some may be reversible)
  - o Wernicke encephalopathy
    - • Demyelination, neuronal loss

Alcohol and The Brain

- Etiology-Pathogenesis-Pathophysiology
  - o Ethanol readily crosses BBB
  - o Neurological damage in alcoholics
    - Direct/indirect EtOH neuro-toxicity
    - Alcohol-related malnutrition
  - o Wernicke encephalopathy
    - Thiamine deficiency impairs dependent enzymes => glutamate accumulation/cell damage
  - o Methanol toxicity
    - Methanol metabolized to formaldehyde, formic acid
    - Causes "anion gap acidosis"
    - Select toxic effect on putamen, optic nerves
    - Commercial products containing methanol include antifreeze, paint remover, photocopying fluid, etc.

Gross Pathologic, Surgical Features
- Wernicke's syndrome
  - o Superior vermis lesions
  - o Mamillary bodies; periventricular midbrain/brainstem
    - Petechial hemorrhage (acute)
    - Mamillary body atrophy (chronic)
  - o Dorsal medial thalamic nuclei (may cause Korsakoff psychosis)
- Corpus callosum atrophy, MS-like WM lesions (chronic EtOH)
- Marchiafava-Bignami disease (callosal necrosis)

Microscopic Features
- Axonal degeneration, demyelination (alcoholic polyneuropathy)
- Purkinje cell loss (alcoholic cerebellar degeneration)

Clinical Issues

Presentation
- Wernicke = triad of ataxia, oculomotor abnormalities, confusion
  - o 80% have polyneuropathy
  - o N.B.: Wernicke can occur in non-EtOH (malnutrition, hyperalimentation, etc)
- Chronic EtOH
  - o Cognitive problems, recent/remote memory impairment
  - o Most common neurologic abnormality = polyneuropathy
  - o Gait abnormalities, nystagmus (cerebellar degeneration)

Natural History
- Ventricular, sulcal enlargement often reversible
- Wernicke encephalopathy: Ocular palsies respond first to thiamine; ataxia, apathy, confusion clear more slowly

Treatment & Prognosis
- Wernicke encephalopathy
  - o Immediate administration of IV thiamine -> quick response
  - o 50% left with slow shuffling gait
- Only 25% of Korsakoff patients achieve full recovery

Selected References
1. Mukamal KJ et al: Alcohol consumption and subclinical findings on magnetic resonance imaging of the brain in older adults. Stroke 32: 1939-46, 2001
2. Comoglu S et al: Methanol intoxication with bilateral basal ganglia infarct. Australas Radiol 45: 357-8, 2001
3. Nutritional And Metabolic Diseases of the Nervous System. Harrisons Online, 380, 1999.

Osmotic Myelinolysis (OM)

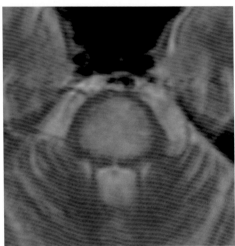

Axial T2WI in a 51-year-old alcoholic male with multiple electrolyte disturbances shows high signal in the central pons. The peripheral fibers are spared. Classic osmotic demyelination.

Key Facts
- Formerly called "central pontine myelinolysis" (CPM)
- 50% in pons but "extra-pontine" myelinolysis (EPM) common
- Heterogeneous disorder with common etiology = osmotic stress
- Osmotic stress = any change in osmotic gradient, not just sodium (e.g., azotemia, hyperglycemia)
- Most common = iatrogenic correction of hyponatremia
- "Co-morbid" conditions common, poorer prognosis

Imaging Findings
<u>General Features</u>
- Confluent symmetric demyelination
- Best diagnostic clue = central pons involved, periphery spared
<u>CT Findings</u>
- NECT: Low density in affected areas (pons, etc.)
- CECT: No enhancement unless very early acute demyelination
<u>MR Findings</u>
- MR >> CT
- N.B.: Variable findings (may be transitory, resolve)
- T1WI
  - Acute: Can be normal/slightly hypointense
  - Subacute: May be hyperintense at 1-4 months
- T2WI, FLAIR
  - Acute: Confluent hyperintensity
  - Subacute: Hyperintensity normalizes
- Contrast: Usually doesn't enhance
<u>Other Modality Findings</u>
- DWI: Restricted (hyperintense)
- ADC: Decreased values
- PET: Early metabolic stress = variable hypermetabolism; late = hypometabolism

Osmotic Myelinolysis (OM)

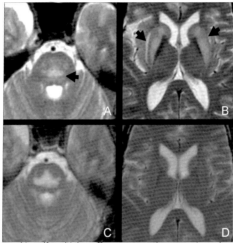

A patient gave himself multiple coffee enemas, then experienced mental status changes. T2WIs show CPM (A, arrow), EPM with bilateral basal ganglia lesions (B, arrows). (C, D) Follow-up shows severe pontine myelinolysis. EPM has resolved.

Imaging Recommendations
- Nonenhanced MR (repeat imaging may be necessary)

Differential Diagnosis
Pontine
- Ischemia, infarction
  - Usually involves **both** central, peripheral pontine fibers
  - Often asymmetric
- Other demyelination (e.g., MS; look for typical lesions elsewhere)
- Neoplasm (e.g., pontine glioma)
  - ADC decreased in CPM

Extrapontine
- Pontine + EPM = almost pathognomonic for OM
- Other demyelination (often asymmetric)
- Other metabolic (Wilson disease, Leigh's)

Pathology
General
- General Path Comments
  - Demyelination without associated inflammation
    - Nonspecific (pattern, distribution suggests OM)
- Etiology-Pathogenesis-Pathophysiology
  - "Osmotic stress" but mechanism of myelinolysis unknown
    - Osmotic insult = change in serum osmolality
    - Relative intracellular hypotonicity
    - Serum osmolality change causes endothelial damage
    - Organic osmolyte deficiency predisposes to endothelial breakdown
    - Endothelial cells shrink, causing BBB breakdown

Osmotic Myelinolysis (OM)

- - Accumulation of hypertonic sodium-rich fluid in ECF
  - Hypertonic ECF, release of myelin toxins damages WM
  - o "Co-morbid" conditions that may exacerbate OM
    - Hepatic, renal, adrenal, pituitary, paraneoplastic disease
    - Nutritional (alcohol, malnutrition, vomiting)
    - Burn, transplantation, other surgical patients
- Epidemiology
  - o Occurs at all ages
  - o Autopsy prevalence varies from <1% to 10%

Gross Pathologic, Surgical Features
- Bilateral/symmetrical, soft, gray-tan discolorations

Microscopic Features
- Extensive demyelination, gliosis
- Macrophages contain engulfed myelin bits and fragments
- Axis cylinders, nerve cells preserved
- No inflammation

Clinical Issues

Presentation
- Often biphasic when hyponatremia present
  - o Initial hyponatremia
    - Seizures, altered mental status, etc
    - Symptoms may resolve with serum osmolality increase
  - o OM symptoms emerge 2-4 days (occasionally weeks) later
    - Changing level of consciousness, disorientation
    - Pseudobulbar palsy, dysarthria, dysphagia (CPM)
    - Movement disorder (EPM)

Natural History
- Spectrum of outcomes
  - o Complete recovery
  - o Minimal residual deficits
    - Memory, cognitive impairment
    - Ataxia, spasticity, diplopia
  - o May progress to
    - Spastic quadriparesis
    - "Locked in"; may progress to coma, death

Treatment & Prognosis
- No consensus; no "optimal" correction rate for hyponatremia
- Self-correction (fluid restriction, discontinue diuretics) if possible
- Plasmapheresis, steroids, glucose infusions being studied

Selected References
1. Cramer SC et al: Decreased diffusion in central pontine myelinolysis. AJNR 22: 1476-9, 2001
2. Waragai M, Satoh T: Serial MRI of extrapontine myelinolysis of the basal ganglia: a case report. J Neurol Sci 161: 173-5, 1998
3. Ho VG et al: Resolving MR features in osmotic myelinolysis (central pontine and extrapontine myelinolysis). AJNR 14: 163-7, 1993

Multiple Sclerosis

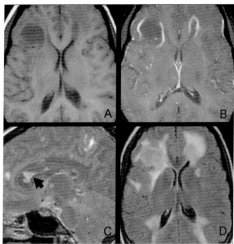

Axial pre- (A) and post-contrast (B) T1WI in a 21- year-old female with MS show lesions with low signal centers, slightly hyperintense rims with partial ring enhancement. FLAIR scans (C, D) show multiple callososeptal lesions (arrow).

Key Facts
- Brain MR abnormal in 95% of patients with clinically definite MS
- "Tumefactive" MS plaque can mimic neoplasm
- Lesion burden on T1WI correlates with clinical disability

Imaging Findings
<u>General Features</u>
- Best diagnostic clues
  - Multiple perpendicular callososeptal hyperintensities
  - Incomplete (semilunar or "horseshoe") rim enhancement

<u>CT Findings</u>
- Iso-/hypodense +/- mild/moderate enhancement

<u>MR Findings</u>
- T1WI
  - Acute: Iso-/mildly hypointense
    - Hypointensity increases in initially demyelinated plaques, decreases in remyelinating lesions
  - Chronic
    - Hypointense center, mildly hyperintense rim ("lesion-within-a-lesion" appearance)
    - Variable atrophy
    - Lesion volume correlates with clinical disability > T2WI
- T2WI, FLAIR (sagittal best)
  - Bilateral, asymmetric linear/ovoid hyperintense lesions
    - Corpus callosum, periventricular region (perpendicular to ventricles, at callososeptal interface)
    - 5% have cortical, 50% subcortical lesions
    - +/- Mass effect/perilesional edema
    - New lesions develop, old often change size
  - Hypointense basal ganglia in 10%-20% of chronic MS cases

Multiple Sclerosis

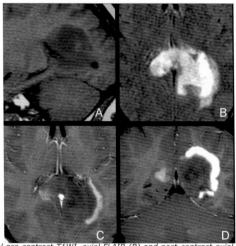

(A) Sagittal pre-contrast T1WI, axial FLAIR (B) and post-contrast axial, coronal (C, D) scans show a solitary "tumefactive" demyelinating lesion of the corpus callosum (courtesy M. Mirfakharee).

- o   Other: Reduced MT; low rCBV (dynamic contrast-enhanced T2*)
- Contrast-enhanced T1WI
  - o   Relative measure of disease activity
  - o   Patterns
    - ▪   Ring > solid
    - ▪   Concentric ("ring-within-a-ring")
    - ▪   Semilunar (incomplete "horseshoe-shaped" rim very suggestive of demyelination)
- Rare: Solitary MS plaque > 4cm, can mimic neoplasm

Other Modality Findings (Vary with Clinical Type)
- MRS: Low NAA, NAA/Cr ratio; elevated Cho; MI, lac variable
- DWI: Increased with bright rim, dark center; elevated ADC in acute

Imaging Recommendations
- Routine MR (sagittal FLAIR, coronal contrast-enhanced T1WI)
- Optional: MRS, DWI

Differential Diagnosis

Acute Disseminated Encephalomyelitis (A.D.E.M.)
- Isolated MS episode difficult to distinguish from A.D.E.M.
- Cortical/subcortical lesions more common in A.D.E.M.

Neoplasm
- Multiple ring-enhancing MS plaques can mimic metastases
- Large, solitary, "tumefactive" MS plaque can mimic glioma

Pathology

General
- General Path Comments
  - o   Findings vary with disease stage
- Etiology-Pathogenesis
  - o   Unknown; probably virus or autoimmune-mediated
  - o   Invasion of activated T cells, microglia attack myelinated axons

Multiple Sclerosis

- Epidemiology
  - Most common cause of CNS demyelinating disease
  - Most common chronically disabling CNS disease in young adults
    - 1 per 1000 in Western world

Gross Pathologic or Surgical Features
- Acute: Poorly-delineated, yellowish-white periventricular plaques
- Chronic: Gray, granular, well-demarcated sunken plaques
- Balo type of MS: Concentric rings of myelinated/demyelinated WM

Microscopic Features
- Perivenous demyelination
  - Active
    - Foamy macrophages with myelin fragments, lipids
    - Reactive astrocytes + inflammatory infiltrates
    - Some lesions hypercellular with atypical reactive astrocytes, mitoses; mimic tumor
  - Chronic
    - Marked loss of myelin, oligodendrocytes
    - Dense gliosis

Clinical Issues

Presentation
- Variable symptoms
  - Acute optic neuritis (50% with +MR will develop MS)
  - Cranial nerve palsy
    - Usually multiple
    - 1%-5% isolated (CNs VI, V most common)
  - Spinal cord symptoms in 80%
- Peak onset = 30y
  - 3%-5% <15y
  - 10% > 50y
- CSF + for oligoclonal bands (absent in 2%-5% of cases)

Natural History
- >80% with "probable" MS, + MR progress to clinically definite MS
- Major clinical subtypes
  - Primary progressive (PP)
  - Secondary progressive (SP)
  - Relapsing-remitting (RR)
- Marburg type MS = clinically fulminant

Treatment & Prognosis
- Steroids, immunotherapy

Selected References
1. Cha S et al: Dynamic contrast-enhanced T2*-weighted MR imaging of tumefactive demyelinating lesions. AJNR 22: 1109-16, 2001
2. Bitsch A et al: A longitudinal MRI study of histopathologically defined hypointense multiple sclerosis lesions. Ann Neurol 49: 793-6, 2001.
3. Mirfakhraee M et al: Semilunar and ring-like enhancing plaques: Imaging features in patients with MS. IJNR 5: 232-9, 1999

Radiation (XRT) and The Brain

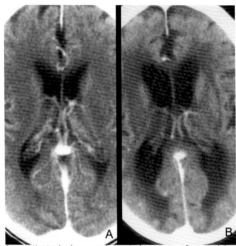

CECT scans in a patient who became demented one year after receiving whole-brain radiation. (A) Initial scan. (B) Follow-up scan shows interval appearance of confluent WM disease, volume loss with enlarged ventricles, sulci.

Key Facts
- CNS XRT has spectrum of pathologic, imaging manifestations
- Includes edema, arteritis, radiation necrosis, mineralizing microangiopathy, progressive leukoencephalopathy, radiation-induced tumors
- Distinguishing residual/recurrent neoplasm from XRT-induced necrosis difficult using morphology alone
- Functional imaging (PET, SPECT) may help

Imaging Findings
General Features
- Radiation injury varies from mild vasogenic edema to frank necrosis
- Periventricular WM especially susceptible
- Best diagnostic sign = hypometabolism, low rCBV on PET/SPECT
CT Findings
- NECT
  - Confluent low density WM within radiation port
  - Basal ganglia/gyriform subcortical Ca++ = mineralizing microangiopathy
- CECT
  - Usually doesn't enhance
  - Necrotizing leukoencephalopathy may have ring-enhancing mass
MR Findings
- Acute: "Fingerlike" WM hyperintense areas on T2WI/FLAIR (vasogenic edema)
- Chronic
  - Radionecrosis of WM
    - Immediate vicinity of tumor/surgical cavity
    - May cause mass effect, can increase in size
  - Most common: Hypointense rim (T2WI), enhances (resembles recurrent/persistent tumor)

Radiation (XRT) and The Brain

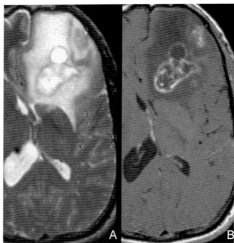

Axial T2WI (A) and post-contrast T1WI (B) in a patient with prior XRT for GBM show left frontal ring-enhancing mass. Biopsy disclosed radiation necrosis without evidence for tumor recurrence.

- ○ Other patterns
  - ▪ Multiple lesions remote from tumor site (nodular, linear, curvilinear, "soap bubble" or "Swiss cheese" enhancement)

<u>Other Modality Findings</u>
- MRS: Low NAA, Cr; Cho 3-4x normal; +/- Lac/Lip peaks
- SPECT, PET: Radionecrosis usually hypometabolic (decreased FDG, methionine, ^{201}Tl uptake), reduced rCBV

<u>Imaging Recommendations</u>
- Contrast-enhanced MR
- PET/SPECT if question of XRT vs. recurrent neoplasm

Differential Diagnosis
<u>Radiation Necrosis vs. Recurrent Neoplasm</u>
- Both often have ring-enhancing mass
- Radionecrosis usually hypometabolic, low rCBV
- Recurrent tumor has high glucose metabolism, Tl uptake with slow washout (N.B.: False-positives have been reported)

<u>Foreign Body Reaction to Hemostatic Materials</u>
- Granulomatous reaction to gelatin sponge, etc.
- Can mimic tumor recurrence, radiation necrosis
- May require biopsy

<u>Tumor/Edema vs. XRT-Induced Demyelination</u>
- Both have WM hyperintensities
- Both may enhance

<u>Radionecrosis vs. Metastasis, Abscess</u>
- MRS helpful

Pathology
<u>General</u>
- General Path Comments
  - ○ Variables include

Radiation (XRT) and The Brain

- Total radiation dose
- Radiation field size
- Radiation fraction size
- Number/frequency of doses
- Adjuvant therapy
- Duration of survival
- Age of patient
  - o Most XRT injury is delayed (months/years)
- Etiology-Pathogenesis
  - o Radiation-induced vascular injury
    - Permeability alterations, endothelial and basement membrane damage
    - Accelerated atherosclerosis
    - Telangiectasia formation
  - o Radiation-induced neurotoxicity
    - Glial and white matter damage (sensitivity of oligodendrocytes >> neurons)
    - Miscellaneous (effects on fibrinolytic system, immune effects)
  - o Rare: Radiation-induced tumor (sarcoma, etc.)
- Epidemiology
  - o Overall incidence of radionecrosis 5%-24%
  - o 5% of those radiated for NP SCCA

Gross Pathologic or Surgical Features
- Spectrum from minor abnormalities to gross cavitating WM necrosis

Microscopic Features
- Vascular changes
  - o Fibrinoid necrosis of blood vessels
  - o Perivascular coagulative necrosis
  - o Wall thickening, hyalinization
  - o Thrombosis, luminal occlusion
  - o Dilated, thin-walled telangiectasias may develop
- White matter changes = focal/diffuse demyelination

Clinical Issues
Presentation
- Highly variable
Natural History
- Radiation-induced necrosis is dynamic pathophysiological process with several possible clinical outcomes
  - o Usually progressive, irreversible
  - o Some lesions stabilize, even regress
Treatment & Prognosis
- Biopsy if imaging doesn't resolve tumor vs. radionecrosis
- Surgery if mass effect, edema

Selected References
1. Chong VF-H et al: Temporal lobe changes following radiation therapy: imaging and proton MRS findings. Eur Radiol 11: 317-24, 2001
2. Kamingo T et al: Radiosurgery-induced microvascular alterations precede necrosis of the brain neuropil. Neurosurg 49: 409-415, 2001
3. Kumar AJ et al: Malignant gliomas: MR imaging spectrum of radiation therapy- and chemotherapy-induced necrosis of the brain after treatment. Radiol 217: 377-84, 2000

CONGENITAL

Chiari I

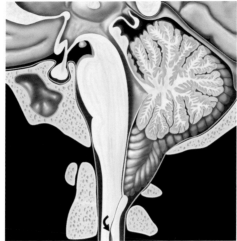

Sagittal graphic depicts Chiari I. Note "peg-like", low-lying tonsil with more vertically-oriented sulci. A collapsed syrinx is illustrated (curved arrow). The 4th ventricle is normal.

Key Facts
- Caused by mild "mismatch" between posterior fossa size (small), cerebellum (normal) => tonsillar "ectopia"
- Tonsils can normally lie below foramen magnum (5 mm or less in adults, slightly more in children <4y)
- Unless tonsils >5mm and/or pointed, probably not Chiari I

Imaging Findings
General Features
- Best diagnostic sign = low-lying, pointed (not round), "peg-like" tonsils with vertical (not horizontal) sulci
- 4th occipital sclerotome syndromes (short clivus, craniovertebral segmentation/fusion anomalies) in 50%
CT Findings
- "Crowded" foramen magnum
- Small/absent PF cisterns
- Lateral/3rd ventricles usually normal
  - +/- Ventriculomegaly
  - Depends upon degree of foramen magnum impaction
MR Findings
- Pointed, triangular-shaped ("peg-like") tonsils
  - ≥ 5mm below foramen magnum **or**
  - Loss of normal round shape
  - Surrounding CSF effaced
- Small bony PF => low torcular, effaced PF cisterns
- Short clivus => apparent descent 4th ventricle, medulla
  - May be real if LP shunt present
- +/- Syringohydromyelia (14%-75%)
Other Modality Findings
- Phase-contrast CSF flow/cord motion MR
  - Demonstrates pulsatile systolic tonsillar descent

Chiari I

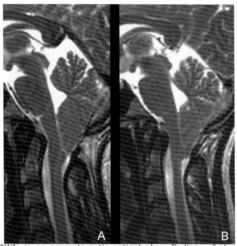

Sagittal T2WIs in an asymptomatic patient show findings of classic Chiari I malformation. Note pointed, "peg-like" tonsils 10 mm below foramen magnum. The tonsillar sulci are oriented almost vertically.

- o Obstructed CSF flow across foramen magnum

Imaging Recommendations
- MR brain +/- CSF flow studies
- Image spine, look for
  - o Syrinx
  - o Low/tethered cord
  - o Fatty filum

Differential Diagnosis
Acquired Tonsillar Ectopia/Herniation
- Basilar invagination
- "Pull from below": LP/LP shunt ⇒ intracranial hypotension with "sagging" brainstem, acquired tonsillar herniation
- "Push from above"
  - o Chronic VP shunt
    - Look for thick skull, premature sutural fusion
    - Arachnoidal adhesions common
  - o Tonsillar herniation 2° ↑ICP, mass effect

Pathology
General
- Genetics
  - o Syndromic/familial
    - Velocardiofacial/microdeletion chromosome 22
    - Williams syndrome
    - Craniosynostosis
- Embryology
  - o Underdeveloped occipital enchondrium ⇒ small posterior fossa vault ⇒ crowded PF ⇒ downward herniated hindbrain ⇒ obstructed

Chiari I

- o   Foramen magnum ⇒ lack of communication between cranial/spinal CSF compartments
- Etiology-Pathogenesis-Pathophysiology
  - o   Hydrodynamic theory of symptomatic Chiari I
    - ▪ Systolic piston-like descent of impacted tonsils/medulla ⇒
    - ▪ **Abnormal** pulsatile intraspinal CSF pressure-wave
    - ▪ May lead to hydrosyringomyelia
- Epidemiology = 0.01% of population

Gross Pathologic, Surgical Features
- Herniated, sclerotic tonsillar pegs; tonsils grooved by opisthion

Microscopic Features
- Purkinje/granular cell loss

Staging or Grading Criteria
- I = asymptomatic: ≈ 14-50%, treatment controversial
- II = brainstem compression
- III = hydrosyringomyelia

Clinical Issues

Presentation
- Up to 50% asymptomatic
- May mimic multiple sclerosis!
- "Chiari I spells": Cough/headache/ sneeze/syncope
- Symptomatic brainstem compression
  - o   Hypersomnolence/central apnea/(infant), sudden death
  - o   Bulbar signs (e.g., lower CN palsies)
  - o   Neck/back pain, torticollis, ataxia
- Symptomatic syringohydromyelia
  - o   Paroxysmal dystonia, unsteady gait, incontinence
  - o   Atypical scoliosis (progressive, painful, atypical curve)
  - o   Dissociated sensory loss/neuropathy (hand muscle wasting)

Natural History
- Increasing ectopia + ↑ time ⇒ ↑ likelihood symptoms
- Children respond better than adults; treat early

Treatment & Prognosis
- Controversial: Intervention for asymptomatic Chiari I + syrinx
- Direct shunting of symptomatic syrinx obsolete
- Aim = restore normal CSF flow at/around foramen magnum
  - o   PF decompression/ resection posterior arch C1
    - ▪ >90% ↓ brainstem signs
    - ▪ >80% ↓ hydrosyringomyelia
    - ▪ Scoliosis arrests (improves in youngest)
  - o   +/- Duraplasty, cerebellar tonsil resection
- Anterior decompression/posterior stabilization rarely indicated (some craniocervical anomalies)

Selected References
1. Genitory L et al: Chiari type 1 anomalies in children and adolescents: Minimally invasive management in a series of 53 cases. Childs Nerv Syst 16(10-11): 707-18, 2000
2. Nishikawa M et al: Pathogenesis of Chiari malformations: A morphometric study of the posterior cranial fossa. J Neurosurg 86: 40-7, 1997
3. Menezes AII: Primary craniovertebral anomalies and the hindbrain herniation syndrome (Chiari 1): Data base analysis. Pediatric Neurosurg 23: 260-69, 1995

Chiari II Malformation (AC2)

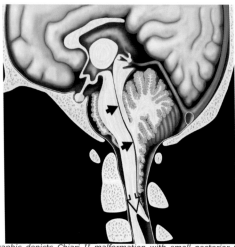

Sagittal graphic depicts Chiari II malformation with small posterior fossa. Note elongated 4ᵗʰ V (arrows). The "cascade" of tissue behind the medulla is the nodulus, choroid plexus, and medullary spur. Open arrow points to the medullary kink. Large massa intermedia, beaked tectum, callosal dysgenesis are illustrated.

Key Facts

- Association with neural tube closure defect (NTD), usually lumbar myelomeningocele (MMC) = virtually 100%
- Small PF ⇒ symptomatic hindbrain herniation/compression
- AC2 most common cause of death in patients with MMC

Imaging Findings

General Features
- Best diagnostic sign = presence of MMC!
- Small PF ⇒ contents shifted down into cervical spinal canal
  - ○ Cerebellar hemispheres/tonsils "wrap" around medulla
  - ○ Pons/cranial nerve roots often elongated
  - ○ Compressed/elongated/low 4ᵗʰ V ⇒ pouch in cervical canal
- Associated abnormalities
  - ○ Dysgenetic CC 90%

CT Findings
- Skull abnormalities
  - ○ "Lacunar" skull (universal at birth, largely resolves by 2y)
    - ▪ Involves inner, outer tables (squamous bones)
    - ▪ Caused by mesenchymal defect, **not** increased ICP
  - ○ Small posterior fossa (PF)
    - ▪ Low lying tentorium/torcular inserts near foramen magnum
    - ▪ Large, funnel-shaped foramen magnum
    - ▪ "Scalloped" petrous pyramid, "notched" clivus
- Dural abnormalities
  - ○ Fenestrated/hypoplastic falx ⇒ interdigitated gyri
  - ○ "Heart-shaped" incisura

MR Findings
- Ventricles
  - ○ Lateral: Pointed anterior horns, colpocephaly

Chiari II Malformation (AC2)

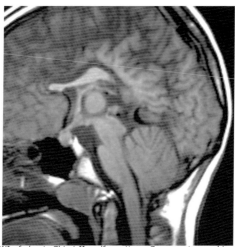

Sagittal T1WI of classic Chiari II malformation. Compare to graphic. Note small posterior fossa, low-lying elongated 4th ventricle, and cascade of tissue behind the medulla. Large massa intermedia, callosal dysgenesis, and malformed gyri are present.

- o 3rd: Large massa intermedia, high-riding if CC agenesis
- o 4th: Elongated, no posterior point (fastigium)
- Small post fossa ⇒
  - o "Towering" cerebellum protrudes up through incisura
    - ▪ Compresses midbrain, causes "beaked" tectum
  - o "Cascade" or "waterfall" of cerebellum/brainstem downwards
    - ▪ Uvula/nodulus/pyramid of vermis ⇒ sclerotic "peg"
    - ▪ Medulla "heaps up" over cord tethered by dentate ligaments ⇒ kink-spur/ "z"-shaped cervico-medullary junction 70%

Other Modality Findings
- Fetal U/S
  - o MMC defined as early as 10 weeks
  - o AC2 ("lemon" and "banana signs") as early as 12 weeks
- MR spine
  - o Open dysraphism, MMC almost 100% (lumbar>>cervical)
  - o Hydrosyringomyelia 20-90%
  - o Posterior arch C1 anomalies 66%
  - o Diastematomyelia 5%

Imaging Recommendations
- Initial screening MR (brain and spine)
- Follow up for
  - o Symptoms of brainstem compression
  - o Increasing ventricular size
  - o Progressive spinal compromise

Differential Diagnosis
Severe, Chronic Shunted Hydrocephalus (Congenital)
- May cause collapsed brain, upward herniated cerebellum

Chiari II Malformation (AC2)

Pathology
General
- General Path Comments
  - Neurogenic renal, orthopedic complications common
- Genetics
  - 4-8% risk recurrence if have one affected child
  - Genetic link to folate deficiency
- Embryology
  - Origins during 4th fetal week
  - Abnormal neurulation $\Rightarrow$ CSF escapes through NTD $\Rightarrow$ failure to maintain 4th ventricular distention $\Rightarrow$ hypoplastic PF chondrocranium $\Rightarrow$ displaced/distorted contents
- Epidemiology
  - 2 to 3:1000 births, decreasing with folate replacement

Gross Pathologic, Surgical Features
- Basic abnormality = herniated hindbrain, hydrocephalus
- Associated abnormalities
  - "Polygyria" with normal 6 layer lamination
  - Heterotopias, (+/-) absent septum pellucidum
  - Aqueduct stenosis

Microscopic Features
- Purkinje cell loss, sclerosis of herniated tissues

Staging or Grading Criteria
- Hydrocephalus, brain malformation relate to
  - Size of PF
  - Degree of caudal descent of hindbrain

Clinical Issues
Presentation
- Fetal screening: $\uparrow$ α-feto protein
- Neonate: MMC, enlarging head, varying degrees of lower extremity paralysis/sphincter dysfunction/bulbar signs

Natural History
- AC2 most common cause of death in MMC
  - Brainstem compression / hydrocephalus
  - Intrinsic brainstem "wiring" defects

Treatment & Prognosis
- Hydrocephalus requires shunting
- Fetal repair MMC in selected patients may ameliorate severity AC2

Selected References
1. Northrup H, Volcik KA: Spina bifida and other neural tube defects. Curr Probl Pediatr 30: 313-32, 2000
2. McLone DG, Naidich TP: Developmental morphology of the subarachnoid space, brain vasculature, and contiguous structures, and the cause of the Chiari II malformation. AJNR 13: 463-82, 1992
3. Friede RL. Ch. 22: Forms of hindbrain crowding, including the Arnold-Chiari malformation. In: Developmental Neuropathology, 2nd ed., 263-276. Springer-Verlag, Berlin 1989

Corpus Callosum (CC) Anomalies

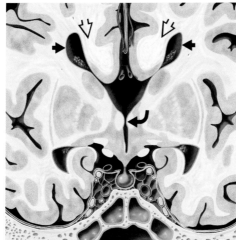

Coronal graphic depicts CC agenesis. Note widely spaced lateral ventricles (black arrows) with "high-riding" 3rd ventricle open dorsally to the interhemispheric fissure (curved arrow). "Probst bundles" (open arrows) are longitudinally oriented white matter (WM) tracts that parallel the insides of the lateral ventricles.

Key Facts
- Most common anomaly seen with other CNS malformations
- One or all segments may be absent (in partial absence, body usually present)

Imaging Findings
General Features
- CC segments front to back = lamina rostralis (unmyelinated), rostrum (myelinated), genu, body, isthmus, splenium
- May be difficult to define prior to myelin maturation
- Best diagnostic signs
  - Axial: Parallel lateral ventricles
  - Coronal: Ventricles resemble "Viking helmet" or "moose head"

CT Findings
- Coronal: High-riding 3rd ventricle
- Axial: Lateral ventricles are key to diagnosis
  - Widely separated, parallel (nonconverging)
  - Persistent fetal shape
    - Occipital horns often dilated (colpocephaly)
    - Pointed anterior horns

MR Findings
- Sagittal
  - High-riding 3rd ventricle (radially arrayed gyri "point to" it)
  - Absent cingulate gyrus
- Coronal
  - "Trident-shaped" anterior horns
  - "Keyhole" temporal horns
  - Vertical hippocampi
  - Probst bundles (longitudinally-oriented white matter tracts)

Corpus Callosum (CC) Anomalies

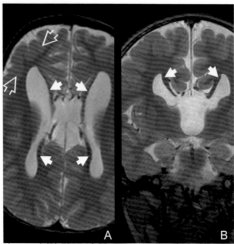

Axial (A) and coronal (B) T2WI of CC agenesis. Note high-riding 3rd ventricle in-between the parallel, nonconverging lateral ventricles. Probst bundles are indicated by the white arrows. Cortical dysplasia is also present (open arrows).

Other Modality Findings
- MRA/MRV
  - "Meandering" or azygous ACAs
  - Persistent falcine sinus

Imaging Recommendations
- MR
  - Other malformations in 50% - 80%
  - Often midline (lipoma, dorsal/interhemispheric cysts, inferior vermian hypoplasia)
  - Cortical maldevelopment (heterotopias, schizencephaly, lissencephaly)
  - Syndromes and sequences (see below)

Differential Diagnosis

Destruction of CC
- Seen with: HIE, infarcts, trauma, surgery
- Findings: CC present, thinned but not shortened

Pathology

General
- Genetics of associated/syndromic CC anomalies
  - Mendelian syndromes, chromosomal anomalies (trisomy 13)
  - Midline anomalies (e.g., DW, Arnold-Chiari)
  - Malformations of the embryonic forebrain occurring prior to CC formation (e.g., holoprosencephaly, frontal encephaloceles)
  - Syndromes/anomalies with mutations in neural adhesion molecules (L1CAM) guiding axonal outgrowth and pathfinding: X-linked CRASH syndrome (CC agenesis, Retardation, Adducted thumbs, Hydrocephalus)

Corpus Callosum (CC) Anomalies

- Embryology
  - CC forms in midline lamina 8-20 weeks
    - Axons form, are guided to midline
    - Callosal growth cones invade posterior lamina terminalis forming CC body
    - Bidirectional growth likely, splenium forms last
    - Growth, elongation, buckling of callosal plate forms genu
    - Anterior lamina terminalis remains thin
- Etiology-Pathogenesis
  - Failure of axons to form (rare, seen only in severe cortical malformations like Cobblestone lissencephaly)
  - Axons aren't guided to midline (mutations in adhesion molecules)
  - Axons reach midline, fail to cross (absence or malfunction of midsaggital guiding "substrate")
  - Axons turn back and form large aberrant longitudinal fiber bundles (Probst bundles) that indent medial ventricular walls
  - Miscellaneous
    - Toxic: Fetal EtOH exposure may affect L1 neuronal cell adhesion molecules
    - Infectious: In-utero CMV
    - Inborn errors of metabolism: Non-ketotic hyperglycinemia, PDH deficiency, maternal PKU, Zellwegers
- Epidemiology
  - 4% of CNS malformations
  - Can be isolated (often males), associated with other CNS malformations

Clinical Issues

Presentation
- Seizures, developmental delay, microcephaly
- Hypertelorism
- Hypopituitarism hypothalamic malfunction

Natural History & Prognosis
- Sporadic/isolated: Normal (especially if partial CC, mild symptoms)
- Complete agenesis + associated/syndromic anomalies = worst

Selected References
1. Kier EL, Truwit CL: The lamina rostralis: Modification of concepts concerning the anatomy, embryology, and MR appearance of the rostrum of the corpus callosum. AJNR 18:715-722, 1997
2. Dobyns, W. B: Absence makes the search grow longer. (Editorial) Am J Hum Genet 58: 7-16, 1996.
3. Kier EL, Truwit CL: The normal and abnormal genu of the corpus callosum: an evolutionary, embryologic, anatomic, and MR analysis. AJNR 17:1631-41, 1996

Dandy-Walker Spectrum (DW)

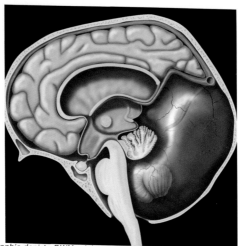

Sagittal graphic depicts DWM. A large CSF-filled cyst extends posteriorly from the 4th ventricular floor. The posterior fossa (PF) is expanded and the torcular Herophili appears markedly elevated. The transverse sinuses descend in a vertical pattern. The vermis is hypoplastic and rotated up/over the cyst.

Key Facts
- DW represents a broad spectrum of cystic PF malformations
- Other anomalies present in most cases

Imaging Findings
General Features of DW Spectrum
- Best diagnostic sign = large PF + big CSF cyst, normal 4th V missing
- DW spectrum (from most to least severe)
  - 4th ventriculocele (10% -15% of cases)
    - Large cyst erodes occipital bone ⇒ "encephalocele" **or**
    - Encysted 4th V herniates into occipital encephalocele
  - "Classic" DW
    - Cystic dilatation of 4th V ⇒ enlarged PF
    - Hypoplastic cerebellum, compressed brainstem
    - Superior vermis remnant rotated up, over cyst
    - High tentorium/venous sinus confluence
  - DW "variant" (mild form of DW complex)
    - Vermian hypoplasia + partial obstruction 4th V
    - Prominent vallecula ("keyhole" appearance)
    - No or small cyst ⇒ PF, brainstem normal
  - Mega cisterna magna
    - Enlarged PF, normal vermis
    - 4th V normal (no cyst, no compression)
    - Cistern **is** crossed by falx cerebelli, tiny veins

CT Findings
- Large posterior fossa
  - Variable-sized cyst
  - Torcular-lambdoid inversion (torcular above lambdoid suture)
  - Occipital bone may appear scalloped, remodeled with all DW types, including mega cisterna magna

Dandy-Walker Spectrum (DW)

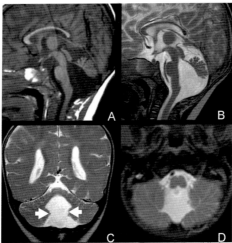

T1- (A) and T2WIs (B-D) show a DW variant. The vermis is mildly hypoplastic and rotated superiorly but the PF is normal size. Note "keyhole" configuration (arrows).

MR Findings
- Sagittal T1WI
  - Floor 4th V present, open dorsally to variable-sized CSF-containing cyst
  - Vermian remnant rotated up, over cyst
  - Elevated torcular with high/steeply sloping tentorium (classic)

Other Modality Findings
- Cyst wall difficult to define without shunt injection

Imaging Recommendations
- MR best characterizes severity, associated anomalies

Differential Diagnosis

Arachnoid Cyst (AC)
- Included in DW spectrum by some authors
- 4th V compressed, displaced but has normal configuration
- AC **not** traversed by falx cerebelli, tiny veins
- ACs lined by arachnoid cells/collagen

Joubert Anomaly
- Episodic hyperpnea, oculomotor apraxia, retinal dystrophy
- Split vermis, "bat-wing" 4thV, mesencephalon shaped like "molar tooth"
- Renal cysts/hepatic fibrosis

Pathology

General
- 2/3rd have associated CNS/extracranial anomalies
  - Craniofacial, cardiac/urinary tract anomalies, polydactyly, orthopedic and respiratory problems
- Genetics (can be sporadic)
  - Syndromic DW occurs with midline defects

Dandy-Walker Spectrum (DW)

- Embryology
  - Common association DW with facial, cardiovascular anomalies suggests onset between formation, migration of neural crest cells (3rd-4th post-ovulatory week)
- Etiology-Pathogenesis-Pathophysiology
  - Hindbrain development arrest
    - Alar plate insult $\Rightarrow$ persistence anterior membranous area
    - 4th V outlet foramina fail to form
    - Straight sinus arrested at vertex (site in fetus)
    - Caudal migration may be mechanically hindered by cyst
- Epidemiology
  - 1:25,000 births
  - Accounts for 1%-4% of all hydrocephalus cases
  - Females $\geq$ males

Gross Pathologic, Surgical Features
- Large PF with big CSF cyst
- Inferior margin vermian remnant continuous with cyst wall
- 4th V choroid plexus absent or displaced into lateral recesses

Microscopic Features
- Outer cyst wall layer continuous with leptomeninges
- Intermediate stretched neuroglial layer is continuous with vermis
- Inner layer of glial tissue lined with ependyma/ependymal nests
- Anomalies of inferior olivary nuclei/corticospinal tract crossings

Staging or Grading Criteria
- Spectrum: 4th ventriculocele (most severe) $\Rightarrow$ Classic DW $\Rightarrow$ DW variant $\Rightarrow$ mega cisterna magna (mildest)

Clinical Issues

Presentation
- 80% diagnosed by 1y (macrocrania, bulging fontanel, etc.)
- Later: Seizures, developmental delay, poor motor skills/balance

Natural History
- Early death common (up to 44%)

Treatment & Prognosis
- CSF diversion: VP shunt (+/-) cyst shunt/marsupialization
- Prognosis depends on supratentorial anomalies, hydrocephalus, related complications
- Intelligence normal in up to 50% of patients with classic DW

Selected References
1. Tortori-Donati P et al: Cystic malformations of the posterior cranial fossa originating from a defect of the posterior membranous area. Mega cisterna magna and persisting Blake's pouch: two separate entities. Childs Nerv Syst 12:303-8,1996
2. Altman NR et al: Posterior fossa malformations. AJR 13: 691-724, 1992
3. Barkovich AJ et al: Revised classification of posterior fossa cysts and cystlike malformations based on the results of multiplanar MR imaging. AJR 153: 1289-1300, 1989

Congenital Lipoma

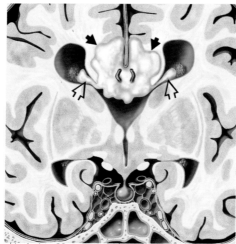

Coronal graphic depicts CC agenesis with interhemispheric lipoma (black arrows). Note intraventricular extension of lipoma through choroid fissures (open arrows). The anterior cerebral arteries are encased by the mass.

Key Facts
- CNS lipomas are congenital malformations, not true neoplasm
- Histologically identical to fat elsewhere in body
- Usually asymptomatic, found incidentally
- Common association between lipoma, corpus callosum (CC) anomalies

Imaging Findings
General Features
- Best diagnostic sign = lobulated extra-axial mass with fat density/ attenuation
CT Findings
- NECT
  - −50 to −100H (fat density)
  - Ca++ varies from none to extensive
    - Rare in posterior fossa, parasellar lesions
    - 65% of bulky tubulonodular CC lipomas
- CECT
  - Doesn't enhance
MR Findings
- Signal intensity identical to fat elsewhere
  - High on T1WI, FSE T2WI, FLAIR
  - Intermediate to high on standard PD (long TR/short TE)
  - Low on standard T2WI
  - Chemical shift artifact (CSA) on conventional PD/T2WI but not FSE
  - Signal suppresses with fat-saturation sequences
- Round/linear "filling defects" present where vessels, cranial nerves pass through lipoma
- May show low signal intensity foci (Ca++)
Other Modality Findings
- U/S: Generally hyperechoic

Congenital Lipoma

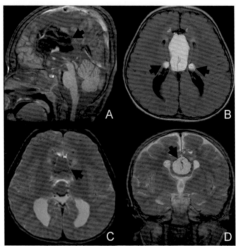

Sagittal fat-suppressed T1WI (A), axial FLAIR (B), axial conventional (C) and corona FSE T2WI (D) show classic agenesis CC with a large tubulonodular interhemispheric lipoma (arrows). The ACAs are encased by the mass. The lipoma extends through the choroid fissures into the lateral ventricles.

<u>Imaging Recommendations</u>
- MR with fat suppression sequence

Differential Diagnosis
<u>Dermoid</u>
- Density usually −20 to −40H
- Signal intensity usually more heterogeneous than lipoma
- Rupture with cisternal fat droplets common
- Usually no associated malformations (common with lipoma)
- Dermoids often calcify; lipomas in locations other than interhemispheric often don't

<u>Teratoma</u>
- Heterogeneous appearance
- Tissue from all 3 embryonic germ layers present
- Contains mucous cysts, fat, chondroid nodules, bony spicules
- Teeth, well-formed hairs rarely present

Pathology
<u>General</u>
- General Path Comments
  - Fat not normally present in CNS
  - Cranial, spinal intradural fat is a congenital anomaly (not a true neoplasm)
  - Size varies from tiny to very large
- Genetics
  - No known defects in sporadic lipoma
  - Occurs in encephalocraniocutaneous lipomatosis, a congenital neurocutaneous syndrome
- Embryology
  - Persistence of embryonic meninx primitiva

Congenital Lipoma

- Normally differentiates into leptomeninges, cisterns
- Maldifferentiates into fat
  - Developing pia-arachnoid invaginates through embryonic choroid fissure (explains frequent intraventricular extension of lipoma)
- Etiology-Pathogenesis-Pathophysiology
  - Congenital malformation
- Epidemiology
  - <0.5% of all intracranial tumors (not true neoplasm)
  - Association with other congenital malformations
    - CC dysgenesis
    - Cephaloceles
    - Closed spinal dysraphism

Gross Pathologic or Surgical Features
- Lobulated fat collection attached to leptomeninges, sometimes adherent to brain
- Cranial nerves, arteries/veins pass through lipoma
- Extra-axial
  - Subarachnoid cisterns (including Meckel cave)
  - May extend into ventricles
- 80% supratentorial
  - Almost half within interhemispheric fissure
    - Thin curvilinear type (along CC body, splenium)
    - Bulky tubulonodular type (frequent Ca++, often associated with CC dysgenesis)
  - Suprasellar 15%-20%
  - 15% quadrigeminal cistern
- 20% posterior fossa (CPA most common site)

Microscopic Features
- Identical to adipose tissue elsewhere
- Cells vary slightly in shape/size, measure up to 200 microns
- Occasional nuclear hyperchromasia
- Mitoses rare/absent
- Liposarcoma = extremely rare malignant intracranial adipose tumor

Clinical Issues

Presentation
- Usually found incidentally at imaging, autopsy

Natural History
- Benign, usually stable
- May expand with corticosteroids
  - High-dose, long-term administration may result in neural compressive symptoms

Treatment & Prognosis
- Generally not a surgical lesion; high morbidity/mortality with little/no benefit
- Reduce/eliminate steroids

Selected References
1. Ickowitz V et al: Prenatal diagnosis and postnatal follow-up of pericallosal lipoma: Report of seven new cases. AJNR 22: 767-72, 2001
2. Bakshi R, Shaikh ZA: MRI findings in 32 consecutive lipomas using conventional and advanced sequences. J Clin Neuroimag 9: 134-40, 1999
3. Truwit CL et al: Pathogenesis of intracranial lipoma: An MR study in 42 patients. AJNR 11: 665-74, 1990

Neuronal Migration Disorders

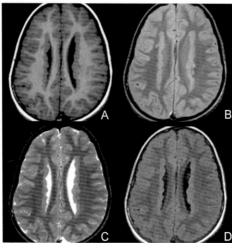

Axial T1WI (A), long TR/short TE (B), T2WI (C) and FLAIR scans show multiple foci of heterotopic gray matter (GM) lining both lateral ventricles. Note "lumpy-bumpy" appearance of the ventricular CSF caused by the heterotopias. The lesions are identical in signal to normal GM. The overlying cortex is slightly thin.

Key Facts
- Neuron migration (germinal zone to cortex) genetically guided
- Arrested/disrupted migration path
  - Can be diffuse or focal
  - Can leave "heterotopic" neuronal deposits anywhere along path
  - Can be inherited or acquired (maternal trauma/infection/toxin)

Imaging Findings
General Features
- Imaging like gray matter (GM)
- Best diagnostic sign = GM "stuck" in wrong place (+/- thin cortex)
CT Findings
- NECT: Always isodense with GM (no Ca++)
- CECT: No enhancement
MR Findings
- Several types (all follow GM on all sequences)
- Described by location, focal/diffuse, anterior/posterior
  - Subependymal heterotopia
    - Most common
    - GM nodules + focal/multifocal indentation of ventricle
  - Subcortical heterotopia
    - Focal/diffuse mass of GM nodules (can mimic neoplasm!)
    - Large foci have thinned overlying cortex, small don't
    - **Or** curvilinear GM mass partially continuous with folded cortex
    - May have abnormal veins
  - Band heterotopia ("double cortex")
    - Thick inner GM band + thin, abnormal cortex (↑ seizure risk)
    - Thin/partial inner band + normal cortex = normal function
  - Lissencephaly type 1 (classic)
    - Thick inner band GM, cell sparse WM zone, thin outer layer GM

Neuronal Migration Disorders

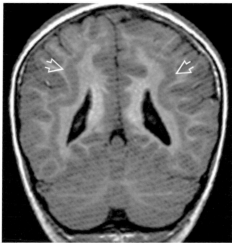

Coronal SPGR illustrates classic laminar ("band") heterotopia (arrows). The overlying appears thinned, especially near the vertex.

- Shallow Sylvian fissure ⇒ brain with "hour-glass" configuration
- Part of agyria, agyria/pachygyria spectrum
  o Lissencephaly type 2 ("cobblestone")
    - Usually occurs with congenital muscular dystrophies
    - Neurons "overmigrate" through gaps in external layer of cortex ⇒ "pebbled" surface of brain
    - Associated ocular, cerebellar anomalies common

Other Modality Findings
- Fetal MR, U/S: Agyric (smooth) cortex normal up to 26 weeks!

Imaging Recommendations
- MRI + thin slice SPGR (surface coil/3D reconstruction) for subtle

Differential Diagnosis

Tuberous Sclerosis
- SENs of tuberous sclerosis may resemble heterotopias
- SENs often calcify, may enhance

Zellweger Syndrome (Peroxisomal Disorder)
- Abnormal neuronal migration, hypomyelination

Pathology

General
- General Path Comments
  o GM nodules/masses in wrong location
- Genetics = complete/partial deletion of genes that govern specific stages of neuronal migration
  o Type 1 (classic or Miller-Dieker) lissencephaly
    - Large deletion LIS1 gene located on 17p13.3
    - Transitory "pioneer cells" arrive first in corticogenesis (layer 1)
    - Migrational failure occurs at multiple stages
  o Isolated lissencephaly/posterior band heterotopia: Smaller deletion LIS1

Neuronal Migration Disorders

- o Isolated lissencephaly/anterior band heterotopia: XLIS gene on Xq22.3-q23
- o Bilateral, diffuse subependymal heterotopia: Filamin-1 gene (required for cell migration to cortex) on Xq28
- Embryology
  - o Subependymal germinal zones proliferate, form neuroblasts, glia
  - o Neuroblasts leave ventricular surface by "leading edge" extension/ growth cone formation (requires filamin)
  - o Neuroblasts attach to radially arranged glial fibers (RGFs)
  - o Neuroblasts migrate along RGFs to mantle (requires cell-adhesion, ligand-receptor interactions)
  - o RGFs guide/nourish migrating neuroblasts
  - o Neuroblasts disengage from RGFs (requires "reelin" secreted by layer 1 pioneer neurons)
  - o Earliest neuroblasts disengage in cortical subplate
  - o Later waves pass through initial layer, form 6-layered cortex
- Etiology-Pathogenesis-Pathophysiology
  - o Genetic: Mutations alter molecular reactions at any/multiple migration points ⇒ migrational arrest, "heterotopic" GM
  - o Acquired: Toxins/infections ⇒ reactive gliosis/macrophage infiltration disturbs neuronal migration/cortical positioning
    - ▪ CMV-infected cells can fail to migrate, cause lissencephaly
    - ▪ Toxins (e.g., EtOH, XRT) ⇒ slow/abnormal migration
- Epidemiology
  - o 17% of neonatal CNS anomalies at autopsy
  - o Found in up to 40% of patients with intractable epilepsy

Gross Pathologic, Surgical Features
- Spectrum: Agyria to normal cortex + small ectopic nodules GM
- Persistent fetal leptomeningeal vascularization if severe

Microscopic Features
- Multiple neuronal cell types, immature/dysplastic neurons
- Neuronal numbers, positioning abnormal

Clinical Issues

Presentation
- Cognitive function, age of seizure onset/severity depends on location/ amount of abnormally positioned GM

Natural History
- Variable life span dependent upon extent of malformation
  - o Type 2 lissencephaly: Months
  - o Focal heterotopias: Can be normal (depends on Sz control)

Treatment & Prognosis
- Resect small accessible epileptogenic nodules
- Corpus callosotomy if bilateral or diffuse unresectable lesions

Selected References
1. Barkovich AJ, Kuzniecky RI: Gray matter heterotopia. Neurology 55: 1603-8, 2000
2. Gressens P: Mechanisms and disturbances of neuronal migration. Pediatric Research 48: 725-30, 2000
3. Hannan Aj et al: Characterization of nodular neuronal heterotopia in children. Brain 122(Pt 2): 219-38, 1999

Neurofibromatosis Type 1 (NF1)

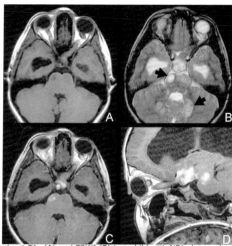

Axial pre-contrast T1- (A) and T2WI (B) in a child with NF1 show enlarged left optic nerve and chiasm with several focal areas of high signal intensity (FASI) in the brainstem and cerebellum (arrows). Some enhancement is present (C, D).

Key Facts
- One of most common inherited CNS disorders
- Most common autosomal dominant disorder
- Most common inherited tumor syndrome

Imaging Findings
General Features
- Focal areas of signal intensity (FASI) in deep GM/WM
- Optic nerve gliomas (ONGs)
- Best diagnostic sign = plexiform neurofibroma (PNF) **anywhere**
CT Findings
- Enlarged optic foramina (ONG) or foramen ovale (PNF)
- Progressive sphenoid wing dysplasia (associated with PNF)
- Lambdoid suture defect
- Dural Ca++ (at vertex)
MR Findings
- FASI
  - Present in 60% of NF1
  - Multiple, non-enhancing lesions with minimal/no mass effect
  - Hyperintense on T2WI, variable T1WI
  - Location: Globus pallidi, WM, thalami, hippocampi, brainstem
  - Pattern: Wax for 2-10 yrs, wane by 20 yrs
  - 11% proliferate: Enhancement, mass effect; excessive numbers, brainstem/splenium/cerebellum
- PNF
  - Orbit/scalp/skull base; paraspinal; other body locations
  - "Target" sign: Bright with central collagen dot on T2WI
- Other Modality Findings
  - MRA/DSA
- Vascular intimal prolifeiation ⇒ stenoses ⇒ moyamoya

Neurofibromatosis Type 1 (NF1)

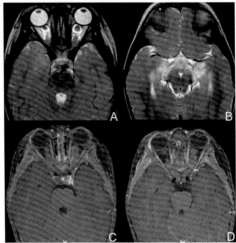

T2- (A, B) and contrast-enhanced T1WIs (C, D) in a child with known NF1 show bilateral enlarged optic nerve sheaths, bilateral ONGs extending posteriorly into the chiasm and retrochiasmatic visual pathway.

- Other: Aneurysms/AVMs; renal artery stenoses, coarctation aorta
- MRS: FASI, tumor both ↑Cho:Cr ratio (tumors higher) but FASI have near normal NAA; tumors show ↓ NAA
- Plain films
  - ○ Scoliosis (often acute angle) 30%
  - ○ Hypoplastic posterior elements, scalloped vertebrae (dural ectasia/ lateral meningoceles > underlying NF)
  - ○ Dysplastic sphenoid wing, ribbon ribs, multiple pseudarthroses

Imaging Recommendations
- Baseline MR brain and orbits +/- spine
- Follow-up if ONG or ↑↑ FASIs

Differential Diagnosis

Other Disorders of the NF Spectrum
- NF2; multiple schwannomatosis syndrome
- Mosaic (segmental) NF1 or NF2
- Hereditary spinal NF
- Familial intestinal NF
- Autosomal dominant café-au-lait spots
- Autosomal dominant neurofibromas alone

Gliomatosis Cerebri (if FASI are extensive)

Pathology

General
- General Path Comments
  - ○ Associated pheochromocytomas, neurofibrosarcomas
- Genetics
  - ○ Autosomal dominant; 50% new mutations
  - ○ Variable expression but virtually 100% penetrance by 5y

Neurofibromatosis Type 1 (NF1)

- o NF gene locus = 17q11.2
- o NF gene product "neurofibromin" is tumor suppressor; inactivation allows tumor development
- Embryology
  - o Disorder of histogenesis
- Etiology-Pathogenesis-Pathophysiology
  - o NF 1 tumor suppressor gene "turned off" in NF1 patients
- Epidemiology
  - o 1:2,500 live births

Gross Pathologic, Surgical Features
- PNF degeneration to neurofibrosarcoma 2-12%
- Visual pathway glioma 15-20%
  - o Symptoms/progression ≤ 5%
  - o Can be isolated (common)/chiasm > extension to geniculate bodies >> postgeniculate tracts
  - o Hamartoma, usually low grade (usual)
  - o Frank malignancy < 20%
  - o Peri-chiasmatic infiltration subarachnoid space
    - ▪ More likely to act aggressively
    - ▪ ↑ Frequency precocious puberty 30%
  - o Dilated optic nerve sheath common (+/- ONG)
- Slight ↑ incidence medulloblastoma/ependymoma
- Definite ↑ incidence astrocytomas
  - o 1-3% of NF1 cases
  - o Earlier presentation, more frequent, more likely multi-centric
  - o Brainstem/cerebellum, splenium CC common sites
    - ▪ Often less aggressive than sporadic brainstem gliomas
    - ▪ But AA, GBM also occur

Microscopic Features
- FASI: Foci of myelin vacuolization
- PNF: Schwann cells, perineural fibroblasts, grow along nerve fascicles

Clinical Issues

Presentation
- NF1 if two or more of the following: ≥ 6 café-au-lait spots (evident during yr 1); ≥ 2 NF [puberty] or 1 PNF; axillary/inguinal freckling; ONG; typical bone lesion; 1° relative with NF
- NF1 related learning disability 30-60%, significant association with hamartomatous changes, esp hippocampal; mental retardation 8%

Natural History
- Cutaneous markers noted later (progressive ↑ conspicuity, number)
- ↑ Incidence MS: Thought due to mutations in oligodendrocyte-myelin glycoprotein gene which is embedded in NF 1 gene

Treatment & Prognosis
- Clinical observation
- Risk other CNS tumors ↑ with presence of ONG
- ↑ Risk sarcomatous degeneration PNF

Selected References
1. Ruggieri M: The different forms of neurofibromatosis. Childs Nerv Syst 15: 295-308, 1999
2. Mukonoweshuro W et al: Neurofibromatosis type 1: The role of neuroradiology. Neuropediatrics 30: 111-19, 1999
3. Gonen O et al: Three-dimensional multivoxel proton MR spectroscopy of the brain in children with neurofibromatosis type 1. AJNR 20: 1333-41, 1999

Neurofibromatosis Type 2 (NF2)

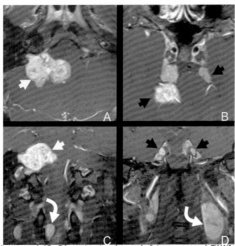

Axial (A, B), coronal (C, D) contrast-enhanced, fat-suppressed T1WI in a patient with NF-2 show a large vestibulocochlear schwannoma (A, C, arrows), bilateral trigeminal schwannomas (B, D, arrows), as well as spinal/paraspinal meningiomas (C, D, curved arrows).

Key Facts
- Autosomal dominant hereditary tumor syndrome with variable expression, 95% penetrance
- Characterized by neoplastic and dysplastic lesions of Schwann, meningeal, and glial cells

Imaging Findings
General Features
- Best diagnostic sign = bilateral vestibular (CN VIII) schwannomas
- Schwannomas of other cranial nerves
- Schwannoma "tumorlets" of spinal nerves common
- Meningiomas (common, often multiple)
- Meningioangiomatosis (rare)
- Intramedullary/conus ependymomas (can be multiple)
- Other lesions: Cerebral calcifications, glial microhamartomas, posterior lens opacities

CT Findings
- NECT
  - Vestibular schwannoma
    - +/- Flared/widened IAC
  - Meningioma
    - High density focal/diffuse dural-based mass(es)
  - Nonneoplastic cerebral Ca++ (usually choroid plexus)

MR Findings
- >95% have CN VIII schwannomas
  - "Ice cream on a cone" mass at/in one or both IACs
    - Iso-/hyperintense on T2WI
    - Strong enhancement
    - Variable cysts, occasionally hemorrhage
- Almost 1/3 have other schwannomas (CN V most common)

Neurofibromatosis Type 2 (NF2)

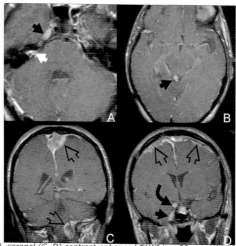

Axial (A, B), coronal (C, D) contrast-enhanced T1WI in a 20 year old with NF2 show multiple schwannomas and meningiomas of the trigeminal (A, D, black arrows), trochlear (B, arrow), oculomotor (D, curved arrow) nerves. Meningiomas (C, D, open arrows), post-surgical changes (A, white arrow) are present.

- 60% meningiomas
  - Diffuse or focal dural enhancement
- Spinal tumors in >90%
  - Ependymoma (cord, conus)
  - Schwannomas (nerve roots, often small/asymptomatic)

Imaging Recommendations
- Contrast-enhanced MR screening of entire neuraxis (brain, spine)

Differential Diagnosis

Multiple Schwannomas Without NF2 ("Schwannomatosis")
- No cutaneous stigmata
- No meningiomas

Pathology

General
- General Path Comments
  - Multiple schwannomas, meningiomas, ependymomas
- Genetics
  - All NF2 families have chromosome 22q12 abnormalities
  - Germline, somatic NF2 gene mutations
    - NF2 functions as tumor suppressor gene
    - Encodes for merlin protein
    - Links cytoskeleton and cell membranes
- Etiology-Pathogenesis-Pathophysiology
  - 50% known family history of NF-2; 50% new mutations
  - Cause truncated, inactivated Merlin protein
  - Loss of both alleles predisposes to tumor formation
- Epidemiology
  - 1 in 40,000-100,000

Neurofibromatosis Type 2 (NF2)

Gross Pathologic, Surgical Features
- See "Schwannoma" and "Meningioma"

Microscopic Features
- NF2-related schwannomas have higher proliferative activity than sporadic tumors but not necessarily more aggressive course

Staging or Grading Criteria
- NF2-associated schwannomas are WHO grade I

Clinical Issues

Presentation
- Clinical diagnosis
  - Bilateral vestibular schwannomas; or
  - 1st degree relative with NF2 and **1** vestibular schwannoma or **2** of the following
    - Meningioma
    - Schwannoma
    - Glioma
    - Neurofibroma
    - Posterior lens opacity, or cerebral calcification
  - Or **2** of the following
    - Unilateral vestibular schwannoma
    - Multiple meningiomas
    - Either schwannoma, glioma, neurofibroma, posterior lens opacity or cerebral calcification
- Most common symptom = hearing loss, vertigo (CN VIII schwannoma)

Natural History
- NF2-associated schwannomas occur earlier in life than sporadic tumors
  - Often multiple
  - Can affect any cranial/peripheral nerve (sensory > motor)

Treatment & Prognosis
- Complete resection of CN VIII schwannoma if feasible
- Subtotal microsurgical resection with functional cochlear nerve preservation in the last hearing ear

Selected References
1. Louis DN et al: Neurofibromatosis type 2. In Kleihues P, Cavanee WK (eds), Tumors of the Nervous System, 216-8, IARC Press, 2000
2. Pollack IF, Mulvihill JJ: Neurofibromatosis 1 and 2. Brain Pathol 7: 823-36, 1997
3. Mautner V-F et al: The neuroimaging and clinical spectrum of neurofibromatosis 2. Neurosurg 38: 880-6, 1996

Tuberous Sclerosis (TSC)

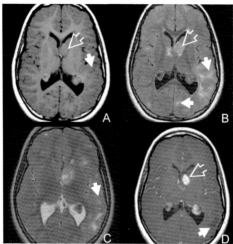

Axial T1WI (A), FLAIR (B), T2WI (C) and contrast-enhanced T1WI in a patient with TSC show cortical tubers with underlying white matter changes (white arrows) and an SGCA at the foramen of Monro (open arrows).

Key Facts
- Inherited tumor disorder with multiorgan hamartomas
- Spectrum of CNS hamartomas, all contain giant balloon cells
- Mutations in TSC tumor suppressor genes cause abnormal cellular differentiation, proliferation

Imaging Findings
General Features
- Best diagnostic sign = 98% have subependymal nodules (SENs)
- Subependymal giant cell astrocytoma (SGCA) 15%
- Cortical/subcortical tubers
- White matter lesions along lines of neuronal migration
- Cortical/subcortical WM lesions 70-95% (variable number)
CT Findings
- NECT
  - SENs
    - Along caudothalamic groove > atrial >> temporal
    - 50% Ca++ (progressive after 1y)
  - Tubers
    - Early: Low density/Ca++ cortical/subcortical mass
    - Later: Isodense/Ca++ (50% by 10y)
  - Ventriculomegaly common even without SGCA
- CECT: Enhancing SEN suspicious for SGCA
MR Findings
- Cortical/subcortical tubers
  - Thickened cortex
    - Pyramidal-shaped gyral expansion
    - 20% have central depression
    - Frontal > parietal > occipital > temporal > cerebellum
  - Variable signal (relative to myelin maturation)
    - FLAIR↑; T1 ↑ or ↓; T2 ↑

Tuberous Sclerosis (TSC)

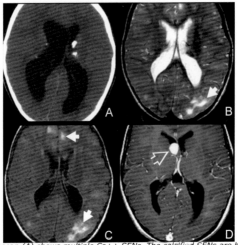

Axial NECT scan (A) shows multiple Ca++ SENs. The calcified SENs are hypointense on T2WI (B). Note cortical tubers, white matter lesions (arrows) on T2WI, FLAIR (C). (D) Contrast-enhanced T1WI shows an SGCA (open arrow).

- ▪ 12% enhance
- White matter (WM) lesions
  - ○ Streaky linear or wedge-shaped hyperintensities (along radial migration lines from ventricle to cortex)
- SENs: Iso or ↑ T1; ↓ T2 and MPGR
  - ○ 30-80% enhance (enlarging SEN at foramen of Munro = SGCA)
  - ○ Other enhancing lesions followed (unless grow, obstruct CSF)
- Focal lacune-like cysts WM (vascular etiology)

Other Modality Findings
- Plain films
  - ○ Bone islands (skull); undulating periosteal new bone (extremity)
- DSA/MRA: Vascular dysplasia (rare = moyamoya, aneurysm)
- PET/SPECT: ↓ Uptake quiescent tubers; ictal SPECT ↑uptake tubers with active Sz focus (helps localize for surgery)
- MRS: ↓ NAA/Cr, ↑ mI/Cr in subcortical tubers, SENs

Imaging Recommendations
- MR with contrast +/- NECT (document Ca++ SENs)

Differential Diagnosis
Taylor's Dysplasia
- Forme fruste of TSC? (single cortical lesion can mimic neoplasm)

X-linked Subependymal Heterotopia
- Isointense to GM T1/T2; don't enhance or Ca++

Pathology
General
- General Path Comments (associated lesions)
  - ○ Renal: Angiomyolipoma and cysts 40-80%
  - ○ Cardiac: Rhabdomyomas 50-65%; majority involute over time
  - ○ Lung: Cystic lymphangiomyomatosis/fibrosis

Tuberous Sclerosis (TSC)

- o   Solid organs: Adenomas; leiomyomas
- o   Skin: Ash leaf spots (majority) including scalp/hair; facial angiofibromas; shagreen patches 20-35% post pubertal; subungual fibromas
- o   Extremities: Subungual fibromas 15-20%; cystic bone lesions; undulating periosteal new bone formation
- o   Ocular: "Giant drusen" (50%)
- o   Dental pitting permanent teeth in most adults with TSC
- • Genetics
  - o   Approximately 50% of TSC cases inherited
  - o   De novo = spontaneous mutation/germ-line mosaicism
  - o   Autosomal dominant, high but variable penetrance
  - o   Two distinct loci: TSC1 (9q34.3) and TSC2 (16p13.3)
- • Etiology-Pathogenesis-Pathophysiology
  - o   Abnormal differentiation/proliferation of germinal matrix cells
  - o   Migrational arrest of dysgenetic neurons
- • Epidemiology
  - o   1:20,000-10,000

Gross Pathologic, Surgical Features
- • Firm cortical masses ("tubers") with dimpling ("potato eye")

Staging or Grading Criteria
- • SGCA = WHO grade I

Clinical Issues

Presentation
- • Diagnostic criteria: Two major or one major/one minor
  - o   Major: Facial angiofibroma/forehead plaque, sub-/periungual fibroma, ≥ 3 hypomelanotic macules, shagreen patch, multiple retinal nodular hamartomas, cortical tuber, SEN, SGCA, cardiac rhabdomyoma, lymphangiomyomatosis, renal angiomyolipoma
  - o   Minor: Dental enamel pits, hamartomatous rectal polyps, bone cysts, cerebral WM radial migration lines (> 3 = major sign), gingival fibromas, nonrenal hamartoma, retinal achromic patch, confetti skin lesions, multiple renal cysts
- • Classic clinical triad
  - o   Facial angiofibromas 90%; retardation 50-80%; Sz 80-90%
  - o   All three = 30%
- • Infant/toddler
  - o   Spasms (65%), autism (50%) bad prognosis
  - o   Occur before development of facial lesions, shagreen patches

Natural History
- • CNS: SCGAs 10-15%

Treatment & Prognosis
- • Resect isolated tubers if seizure focus if multiple lesions
- • SGCAs resected if obstructing foramen of Monro

Selected References
1.   Braffman B, Naidich TP: The phakomatoses: Part 1: Neurofibromatosis and tuberous sclerosis. Neuroimag Clin N Amer 4:299-324, 1994
2.   Roach ES et al: Tuberous sclerosis complex consensus conference: Revised clinical diagnostic criteria. J Child Neurol 13: 624-28, 1998
3.   Griffiths PD, Martland TR: Tuberous sclerosis complex: The role of neuroradiology. Neuropediatrics 28: 244-52, 1997

Sturge-Weber Syndrome (SWS)

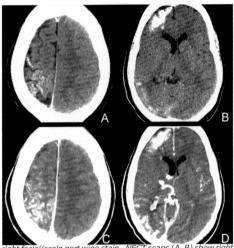

Patient with right facial/scalp port wine stain. NECT scans (A, B) show right hemisphere atrophy, gyriform cortical Ca++, and ipsilateral calvarial thickening. (C, D) CECT scans show enhancing pial angioma, prominent choroid plexus and enlarged collateral deep venous drainage channels.

Key Facts
- "Port wine stain" facial nevus
- Also known as encephalotrigeminal angiomatosis
- Usually a sporadic congenital (but not inherited) malformation
- Fetal cortical veins fails to develop normally
- Imaging sequelae caused by chronic venous ischemia

Imaging Findings
General Features
- Findings relate to sequelae of progressive venous occlusion
- Best diagnostic sign = cortical Ca++/atrophy + enlarged choroid plexus
CT Findings
- NECT
  - Gyral/subcortical WM Ca++
    - Ca++ **not** in leptomeningeal angioma
    - Progressive, generally posterior to anterior (2-20y)
  - Late
    - Atrophy
    - Hyperpneumatization paranasal sinuses
    - Thick diploe
- CECT
  - Serpentine leptomeningeal enhancement
  - Ipsilateral choroid plexus enlargement almost universal
MR Findings
- Early: "Accelerated" myelin maturation 2° transient hyp**er**perfusion
  - Pial angioma, subarachnoid space vessels/trabeculae enhance
- Late: "Burnt-out"⇒ ↓ pial enhancement, ↑ cortical/subcortical Ca++; atrophy, white matter gliosis (↑ signal T2)

Sturge-Weber Syndrome (SWS)

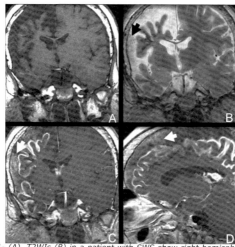

Coronal T1- (A), T2WIs (B) in a patient with SWS show right hemisphere atrophy, subcortical Ca++. Coronal (C) and sagittal (D) contrast-enhanced T1Wis show the pial angioma enhances intensely. Note enhancing trabeculae in SAS (arrows).

<u>Other Modality Findings</u>
- DSA: Pial blush, paucity of normal cortical veins
- MRV
  - Lack superficial cortical veins
  - ↓ Flow transverse sinuses/jugular veins
  - ↑↑ Prominence deep collateral (medullary/subependymal) veins
  - Progressive sinovenous occlusion
- PET: Progressive hypoperfusion/glucose hypometabolism
- MRS: ↓ NAA in affected areas
- SPECT: Transient hyperperfusion (early)
- Orbital enhancement > 50%

<u>Imaging Recommendations (N.I.H.)</u>
- MR with contrast (assess extent, uni-/bilaterality, orbital involvement)

Differential Diagnosis
<u>Other Vascular Phakomatoses (Neurocutaneous Syndromes)</u>
- Wyburn-Mason syndrome
  - Facial vascular nevus
  - Visual pathway and/or brain AVM
- Klippel-Trenaunay-Weber syndrome
  - Osseous/soft-tissue hypertrophy, extremity vascular malformations
  - May be combined with some features of SWS
- Meningioangiomatosis
  - Ca++ common; variable leptomeningeal enhancement
  - May invade brain through VRSs
  - Atrophy usually absent

<u>Celiac Disease</u>
- Bilateral occipital Ca++
- Predominantly Mediterranean (Italian) ancestry
- No angiomatous involvement brain/face

Sturge-Weber Syndrome (SWS)

Pathology

<u>General</u>
- General Path Comments
  - Cutaneous nevus flammeus CN V_1
  - +/- Visceral angiomatosis
- Genetics
  - Usually sporadic with no known inheritance
  - Very rare: Familial or with other vascular phakomatosis
- Embryology
  - Embryonic cortical veins fail to coalesce, develop
  - Persistence of primordial vessels
    - Occurs at 4-8 week stage
    - Visual cortex adjacent to optic vesicle and upper fetal face
- Etiology-Pathogenesis-Pathophysiology
  - Arrested development fetal vasculature $\Rightarrow$ deep venous occlusion, venous stasis $\Rightarrow$ anoxia cortex
- Epidemiology
  - Rare: 1:50,000

<u>Gross Pathologic, Surgical Features</u>
- Meningeal hypervascularity/angiomatosis
- Subjacent cortical/subcortical Ca++

<u>Microscopic Features</u>
- Pial angioma = multiple thin-walled vessels in enlarged sulci
- Cortical atrophy, Ca++

Clinical Issues

<u>Presentation</u>
- CN V_1 facial nevus flammeus ("port wine stain") 98%
- Pial angiomatosis unilateral 80%, bilateral 20%
  - Seizures 90%; hemiparesis 30 – 66%
  - Stroke-like episodes; neurological deficit 65%
- Eye findings esp. with upper and lower lid nevus flammeus
  - Choroidal angioma 70% $\Rightarrow$ ↑ intraocular pressure/ congenital glaucoma $\Rightarrow$ buphthalmos
- Retinal telangiectatic vessels; scleral angioma; iris heterochromia
- Seizures (Sz) develop first year of life
- Infantile spasms $\Rightarrow$ tonic/clonic, myoclonic
  - If Sz $\Rightarrow$ developmental delay 43%, emotional/behavioral problems 85%, special education 70%, employability 46%
- Progressive hemiparesis 30%, homonymous hemianopsia 2%

<u>Natural History</u>
- Progressive sz, neurological deficit, atrophy

<u>Treatment & Prognosis</u>
- ↑ Extent of lobar involvement, white matter alterations, and degree of atrophy $\Rightarrow$ ↑ likelihood Sz (also developmental delay)

Selected References
1. Maria BL et al, Central nervous system structure and function in Sturge-Weber syndrome: Evidence of neurologic and radiologic progression. J Child Neurol 13: 606-18, 1998
2. Sujansky E, Conradi S. Outcome of Sturge-Weber syndrome in 52 adults. Am J Med Genet 22; 57: 35-45, 1995
3. Braffman B, Naidich TP. The Phakomatoses: Part II. Neuroimaging Clinics of North America 4: 325-48, 1994

Von Hippel-Lindau Disease (VHL)

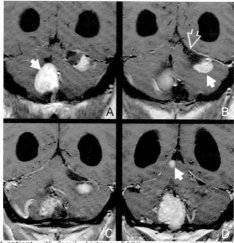

34-year-old patient with family history of VHL presents with headache. Coronal contrast-enhanced T1WIs show 3 cerebellar hemangioblastomas (white arrows). Note cystic component (open arrows).

Key Facts
- Autosomal dominant hereditary tumor syndrome with high penetrance, variable expression
  - Affects six different organ systems, including eye and CNS
  - Involved tissues often have multiple lesions
  - Lesions = benign cysts, vascular tumors, carcinomas
- Phenotypes based on absence or presence of pheochromocytoma
  - Type 1 = without pheochromocytoma
  - Type 2A = with both pheochromocytoma, renal cell carcinoma
  - Type 3A = with pheochromocytoma, without renal cell carcinoma

Imaging Findings
General Features
- Varies with organ, lesion type
- Best diagnostic sign = 2 CNS hemangioblastomas or 1 + retinal hemorrhage

CT Findings
- NECT
  - 2/3 well-delineated cerebellar cyst + nodule, 1/3 solid
  - +/- Obstructive hydrocephalus
- CECT
  - Intense enhancement

MR Findings
- Contrast-enhancing nodule + cyst or syrinx (cord)
- May detect tiny enhancing nodules

Other Modality Findings
- DSA shows intensely vascular mass, prolonged stain

Imaging Recommendations (N.I.H.)
- Contrast-enhanced MR of brain/spinal cord from age 11y, every 2 years
- U/S of abdomen from 11y, yearly

Von Hippel-Lindau Disease (VHL)

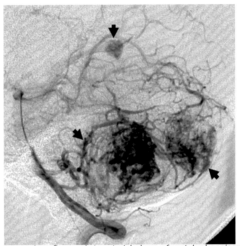

Same case as previous figure. Late arterial phase of vertebral angiogram, lateral view, shows the 3 hemangioblastomas are intensely vascular (arrows).

- Abdominal CT from 20y, yearly or every other year
- MRI of temporal bone if hearing loss, tinnitus/vertigo

Differential Diagnosis
Pilocytic Astrocytoma (Cerebellum)
- Different age (usually younger)
Metastasis
- Usually solid, not cyst + nodule
- Some tumors (e.g., renal clear cell carcinoma) can resemble hemangioblastoma histopathologically

Pathology
General
- General Path Comments
  - VHL characterized by development of
    - Capillary hemangioblastomas of the CNS and retina
    - Cysts, renal cell carcinoma
    - Pheochromocytoma
    - Pancreatic cysts, islet cell tumors
    - Inner ear (endolymphatic sac) tumors
    - Epididymal cysts, cystadenomas
- Genetics
  - Autosomal dominant inheritance
  - Germline mutations of VHL tumor suppressor gene
    - Chromosome 3p25-26
    - Involved in cell cycle regulation, angiogenesis
    - Different mutations scattered throughout gene
    - Disease features vary depending on specific VHL mutations
    - Inactivating mutations (nonsense mutations/deletions) predispose to VHL type 1
    - Missense mutations predispose to VHL types 2A, 2B

Von Hippel-Lindau Disease (VHL)

- Etiology-Pathogenesis-Pathophysiology
  - Both alleles of tumor suppressor gene inactivated
  - Suppressor gene product = VHL protein
  - Mechanism by which neoplasia is induced unclear
- Epidemiology
  - 1 in 35-50,000 (no racial, gender predilection)
  - 25% of capillary hemangioblastomas associated with VHL

Gross Pathologic, Surgical Features
- Well-circumscribed, very vascular, reddish nodule
- 75% at least partially cystic, contain amber-colored fluid

Microscopic Features
- Two components
  - Rich capillary network
  - Large vacuolated stromal cells with clear cytoplasm
- Immunohistochemistry = for cytokeratins, Lu-5

Staging or Grading Criteria
- Capillary hemangioblastoma = WHO grade I

Clinical Issues

Presentation
- Clinically heterogeneous; phenotypic penetrance = 97% at 65y
- Diagnosis of VHL = capillary hemangioblastoma in CNS/retina *and* one of typical VHL-associated tumors *or* previous family history
- Hemangioblastomas usually occur in adults
  - Retinal
    - Mean age = 25y
    - Visual symptoms (retinal detachment, vitreous hemorrhage)
  - Cerebellar
    - Mean age = 30y
    - H/A (obstructive hydrocephalus)
  - Spinal cord
    - Progressive myelopathy (tumor + syrinx)
- VHL-associated tumors
  - Pheochromocytoma (30y)
  - Renal carcinoma (33y)
  - Endolymphatic duct tumor

Natural History
- Renal carcinoma proximal cause of death in 15%-50%

Treatment & Prognosis
- Ophthalmoscopy yearly from infancy
- Physical/neurological examination, from 2y, yearly
- Surgical resection of symptomatic cerebellar/spinal hemangioblastoma
- Stereotactic radiosurgery may control smaller lesions
- Laser treatment of retinal angiomata

Selected References
1. Bohling T et al: Von Hippel-Lindau disease and capillary hemangioblastoma. In Kleihues P, Cavanee WK (eds): Tumours of the Central Nervous System, 223-6, IARC Press, 2000
2. Hes FJ, Feldberg MAM: Von Hippel-Lindau disease: strategies in early detection (renal-, adrenal-pancreatic masses). Eur Radiol 9: 598-610, 1999
3. Neumann HPH et al: Von Hippel-Lindau syndrome. Brain Pathol 5: 181-93, 1995

Myelin Maturation

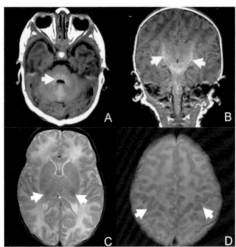

Axial T1WI (A), coronal SPGR (B), and axial T2WI (C, D) show normal myelination at age 2 weeks. Only the dorsolateral midbrain (A, arrow) and posterior limb of internal capsule (B, C, arrows) are myelinated. The perirolandic cortex normally appears hypointense on T2WI (D, arrows).

Key Facts
- Oligodendrocytes form, maintain axon myelin sheath
- One oligodendrocyte may invest up to 50 axons
- Normal myelination begins at 16 weeks gestational age ⇒ nearly complete by 2 years
- Maturation proceeds caudal to rostral, central to peripheral, dorsal to ventral, in order of need (perirolandic gyri, visual cortex early)

Imaging Findings
General Features
- Imaging reflects lipid/water content/myelinated fiber density
- Know gestational age before assigning myelination stage!
CT Findings
- NECT: Unmyelinated WM appears very low density
MR Findings
- Myelination precursors and progressive myelin maturation ⇒ T1 / T2 shortening (↑ signal T1, ↓ signal T2)
  - ↑ Cholesterol/glycolipids of forming myelin
  - Spiraling/myelin compaction causes ↓ H_2O content
- Progressive T1/T2 shortening continues through teens
- Heavy myelination, high density of compact fiber bundles (anterior commissure, corpus callosum, forniceal columns, Probst bundles) ⇒ very bright T1, very dark T2
- T1 lags weeks behind histological myelin maturation assessment: Minimal concentration myelin needed to allow visualization
- Lower concentration myelin needs to be seen on T1WI; maturation on T2WI lags by 2 - 4 months
Other Modality Findings
- DWI: ADC values predate T1/T2-weighted signal changes

Myelin Maturation

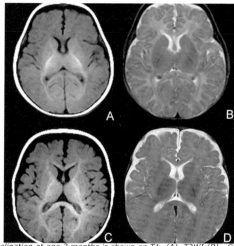

Normal myelination at age 3 months is shown on T1- (A), T2WI (B). Compare with normal myelination at age 7 months (C, D). Much of the central white matter, including the corpus callosum, is densely myelinated.

- ^{123}I-IMP SPECT /PET: ↑ Relative rCBF /metabolic rates in areas of maturing myelin
- Magnetization transfer: ↑ Mean MTR with brain myelination

Imaging Recommendations
- MRI with both T1-, T2-weighting; IR may replace T1
- T1, IR more sensitive to 8 months
- T2 more sensitive after 8 months
- Myelin "looks older" on FSE T2WI (know your sequences!)
- Image during window of opportunity (3y or earlier)

Differential Diagnosis
Dysmyelinating Diseases
Demyelinating Diseases

Pathology
General
- General Path Comments
  - Disorders of CNS myelin (oligodendroglia), PNS myelin (Schwann cells) may occur together
- Genetics (myelin maturation)
  - Chr 18q governs myelin basic protein (MBP)
  - Other chromosomes also involved in myelin synthesis
- Embryology
  - Oligodendrocyte precursors proliferate in germinal matrix
  - Adhesion molecules (neural cell adhesion molecule, NCAM) bring axon and glial cell together; transduce electrical impulse
  - Neuron induces myelinization by electrical impulse
  - Myelin presence inhibits oligodendrocyte progenitor maturation ⇒ immature cells persist in adult CNS to restore damaged myelin

Myelin Maturation

- Etiology-Pathogenesis-Pathophysiology
  - Myelin delay (numerous chromosomal anomalies)
  - Some associated with deletion/mutations of genes governing myelin proteins $\Rightarrow$ abnormal myelin structure
    - Autosomal, X-linked mutations may affect oligodendrocytes
    - Adhesion/regulatory cell mutations $\Rightarrow$ abnormal myelination
  - Pelizaeus-Merzbacher
    - Mutations proteolipid protein (PLP) gene (located Chr Xq22)
  - Other disorders affecting myelin
    - Myelin breakdown (inflammation, inborn errors of metabolism)
    - Thyroid hormone needed for oligodendrocyte proliferation and maturation
    - Hypermyelination: Hypoxic-ischemic encephalopathy (HIE) $\Rightarrow$ status marmoratus of basal ganglia/thalami

Gross Pathologic, Surgical Features
- Pre myelinated brain "soft" due to higher H20 content

Microscopic Features
- Myelination "gliosis" is normal, − massive proliferation of glial cells before onset myelination, not the same as "reactive gliosis"
- HIE damage occurs in areas of actively myelinating brain ($\uparrow$ metabolic activity)

Staging or Grading Criteria
- Milestones on T1WI
  - Birth: Dorsal brainstem, central CBLL WM, posterior limb internal capsule, lateral thalamus, corona radiata to para-Rolandic stripe
  - 1 month: Anterior limb internal capsule, optic radiations
  - 3 months: Belly of pons, CBLL folia
  - 4-8 months: Progressive myelination CC, centrum semiovale
  - 8 months: Peripheral arborization, adult extent although not adult fullness on T1
- "Lag" in T2WI: "Crossover" (from infantile to adult signal) occurs between 6 months and 2y
  - 18 months: Adult fullness on T1-, adult extent on T2WI
  - 3 years: Peripheral WM arborization (temporal, frontal poles)
  - After 3 years: WM "bulks up" to adult appearance on T2WI

Clinical Issues

Presentation
- Clinical symptoms vary according to cause of myelin delay

Natural History
- +/- Slow catch up of myelin milestones may occur

Treatment & Prognosis
- Treatment for myelin delay occasionally possible (thyroid deficiency, B12 deficiency)

Selected References
1. Barkovich AJ: Concepts of myelin and myelination in neuroradiology. AJNR 21: 1099-1109, 2000
2. Nakagawa H et al: Normal myelination of anatomic nerve fiber bundles: MR analysis. AJNR 19: 1129-36, 1998
3. Van der Knaap MS, Valk J: Chapter 1 Myelin and white matter. In: Magnetic resonance of myelin, myelination, and myelin disorders, 1-17, 2nd ed. Springer, Berlin, 1995

Inherited Metabolic Disorders

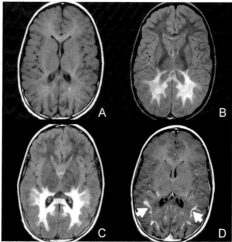

T1WI (A), PD (B), FLAIR (C) scans of X-linked ALD show symmetric periatrial, splenium lesions. The rim of active demyelination enhances (D, arrows).

Key Facts
- Abnormal gene/enzyme ⇒ metabolic blockade ⇒ cell malfunction
  - Accumulation of toxic intracellular substrate **or**
  - Deficiency of necessary product or metabolite
- Three organelles with three major disorders
  - Lysosomes ("garbage collector"): Mucopolysaccharidoses (MPS)
  - Peroxisomes (myelin formation/stabilization): X-linked adrenoleukodystrophy (ALD)
- Mitochondria (cell's "power house"): Leigh disease

Imaging Findings
General Features
- Patterns of "selective vulnerability"
  - Appearance depends upon
    - Amount of residual enzyme
    - Stage of brain development
    - Sensitivity of various cells to type of insult
- Best diagnostic signs: Look for symmetry, geographic patterns, involvement of specific nuclei/tracts, enhancement
  - Centrifugal (inside to outside) spread most common, nonspecific
  - Frontal vs. posterior (ALD posterior)
  - Enhancement (ALD yes, MLD no)
  - Specific nuclei (e.g., putamen with Leigh)
  - Preferential involvement
    - WM, GM or both
    - Sub-cortical "U" fibers/deep WM/cerebellum
- Caveats
  - Distinguishing WM vs. GM not always possible on imaging alone!
  - Beware demyelination from any cause (e.g., HIE)
  - Neuron dies ⇒ axons degenerate, demyelinate ("leukodystrophy")

Inherited Metabolic Disorders

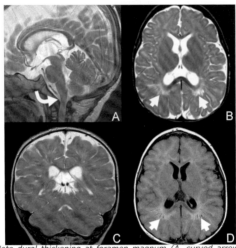

MPS 1. Note dural thickening at foramen magnum (A, curved arrow), enlarged perivascular spaces (PVSs, B-D, arrows).

<u>CT Findings (Most Common Features, Common Disorders)</u>
- Leigh: Symmetrical ↓ density BG/thalami
- MPS: Macrocrania, "Hurler's holes" (enlarged PVSs)
- X-ALD: ↓ Density splenium/posterior WM +/- Ca++

<u>MR Findings</u>
- Leigh: Symmetrical ↑ T2 putamen/caudate, periaqueductal GM
- MPS: Dilated PVSs, progressive hydrocephalus **and** atrophy
- X-ALD: Demyelination begins splenium ⇒ peritrigonal WM ⇒ corticospinal tracts/fornix; leading edge enhances

<u>Other Modality Findings</u>
- MRS: ↓ NAA (non-specific) or documents typical spectra
  - Lactate peak with mitochondrial disease
  - Active X-ALD: ↓ NAA; ↑Cho, MI, lactate

<u>Imaging Recommendations</u>
- Baseline MRI/MRS; f/u complications, therapeutic response

Differential Diagnosis
<u>Leigh</u>
- Wernicke encephalopathy (history of ETOH or nutritional deficiency; mammillary bodies involved)
- Reversible striatal necrosis (see "ADEM")

<u>MPS</u>
- Macrocephaly with dilated VRSs
- <u>X-ALD</u>
- MLD (may involve the splenium/peritrigonal WM, doesn't enhance)

Pathology
<u>General</u>
- General Path Comments
  - Leigh
    - Growth failure, liver failure, heart block/cardiomyopathy

- o MPS: Glycosaminoglycans accumulate in most organs/ligaments
  - ▪ Hepatosplenomegaly, arterial wall thickening
  - ▪ Dural thickening (cord compression at foramen magnum)
  - o X-ALD: Skin bronzing, adrenal failure
- • Genetics (myelin maturation)
  - o Leigh: Autosomal recessive/maternal inheritance
  - o MPS: Autosomal recessive (exception: X-linked MPS 2)
  - o X-ALD: X-linked recessive (10-20% female carriers)
- • Etiology-Pathogenesis-Pathophysiology
  - o Leigh: Mitochondrial failure ⇒ cellullar energy failure
  - o MPS: Ganglioside accumulation (especially toxic to neurons)
  - o X-ALD: Peroxisomal deficiency ⇒ very long chain fatty acids accumulate ⇒ brittle myelin
- • Epidemiology: All are **rare!**

Gross Pathologic, Surgical Features
- • Leigh: Ischemia (regions of high metabolic demand)
- • MPS: Thick meninges, dilated VRSs ("cribiform" appearance)
- • X-ALD: Atrophy, WM softened (posterior early, diffuse late)

Microscopic Features
- • Leigh
  - o Spongiosis, astrogliosis
  - o Demyelination, capillary proliferation
- • MPS: Glycosaminoglycans accumulate in dilated V-R spaces
- • X-ALD
  - o Complete myelin loss ("U" fibers preserved), astrogliosis
  - o Ca++ (late), prominent inflammatory changes

Clinical Issues

Presentation
- • Age at onset/symptoms/progression depend on amount of residual enzyme present
  - o Severe deficiency ⇒ infant, often multi-organ, rapid course
  - o Near-normal levels ⇒ late childhood/adult, slowly progressive
- • Leighs
  - o Multisystem energy failure
  - o CNS: Developmental delay, loss of milestones, seizures
- • MPS: Typical facies, joint contractures, hepatosplenogmegaly
- • X-ALD
  - o Pre-teen male with skin bronzing
  - o Behavioral/learning difficulties
  - o Progresses to spastic quadriparesis, blind, deaf

Natural History
- • Rate of progression depends upon amount residual enzyme

Treatment & Prognosis
- • MPS, X-ALD: Bone marrow transplant may be option
- • Leigh: Co-enzyme Q, riboflavin/vitaminC/menadione may help

Selected References
1. Van der Knaap MS, Valk J: Chapter 3: Selective vulnerability. In: Magnetic Resonance of Myelin, Myelination, and Myelin Disorders, 2nd ed, 22-30, Springer, 1995
2. Barkovich AJ: Concepts of myelin and myelination in neuroradiology. AJNR 21: 1099-1109, 2000
3. Blaser SI et al: Neuroradiology of lysosomal disorders. Neuroimaging Clin N Amer 4:283-298, 1994

Index of Diagnoses

NOTES

NOTES

NOTES

NOTES

NOTES

NOTES

NOTES